NURSING RESEARCH USING LIFE HISTORY

Mary de Chesnay, PhD, RN, PMHCNS-BC, FAAN, is professor and immediate past-director of WellStar School of Nursing, Kennesaw State University, Georgia, as well as a licensed psychotherapist and a nurse–anthropologist researcher. In her private psychotherapy practice (active practice since 1973), Dr. de Chesnay has specialized in treating sexually abused and trafficked children, has developed culturally based interventions, and has taught content about vulnerable populations for many years. The third edition of Dr. de Chesnay's book, *Caring for the Vulnerable,* was published in 2012. She has authored six book chapters and 19 journal articles. She is principal investigator (PI) or co-PI on numerous grants and has served as a consultant on research, academic, continuing education, and law enforcement projects. Recently, Dr. de Chesnay was invited to serve on the Georgia State Governor's Task Force called CSEC (Commercial Sexual Exploitation of Children). She has presented nationally and internationally in nursing and anthropology, and has published on incest and sex tourism and about applying various qualitative approaches to clinical research. She has been invited as a keynote speaker at numerous conferences including Sigma Theta Tau and the International Society of Psychiatric Nurses.

Nursing Research Using Life History

Qualitative Designs and Methods in Nursing

Mary de Chesnay, PhD, RN, PMHCNS-BC, FAAN

Editor

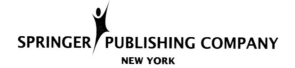

SPRINGER PUBLISHING COMPANY

NEW YORK

Springer Publishing Company, LLC
11 West 42nd Street
New York, NY 10036
www.springerpub.com

Acquisitions Editor: Joseph Morita
Production Editor: Brian Black
Composition: Exeter Premedia Services Private Ltd.

ISBN: 978-0-8261-3463-9
e-book ISBN: 978-0-8261-3464-6

14 15 16 17 / 5 4 3 2 1

The author and the publisher of this Work have made every effort to use sources believed to be reliable to provide information that is accurate and compatible with the standards generally accepted at the time of publication. The author and publisher shall not be liable for any special, consequential, or exemplary damages resulting, in whole or in part, from the readers' use of, or reliance on, the information contained in this book. The publisher has no responsibility for the persistence or accuracy of URLs for external or third-party Internet websites referred to in this publication and does not guarantee that any content on such websites is, or will remain, accurate or appropriate.

Library of Congress Cataloging-in-Publication Data
Nursing research using life history : qualitative designs and methods in nursing / Mary de Chesnay, editor.
    p. ; cm.
    Includes bibliographical references.
    ISBN 978-0-8261-3463-9—ISBN 978-0-8261-3464-6 (e-book)
    I. De Chesnay, Mary, editor.
    [DNLM: 1. Nursing Research—methods. 2. Autobiography as Topic. 3. Interviews as Topic.
    4. Qualitative Research. WY 20.5]
    RT81.5
    610.73072—dc23
                                                                                2014007676

Printed in the United States of America by Gasch Printing.

For my cousin, Sue Dagit, a woman of substance, compassion, and integrity.

—MdC

CONTENTS

Contributors

Joan L. Bottorff, PhD, RN, FCAHS, FAAN, is professor of nursing at the University of British Columbia, Okanagan campus, faculty of Health and Social Development. She is the director of the Institute for Healthy Living and Chronic Disease Prevention at the University of British Columbia.

Brenda Brown, RN, BSN, MS, CNE, is an assistant professor of nursing at Brenau University and a doctoral student at Kennesaw State University. She is the treasurer of the Nu Gamma chapter of Sigma Theta Tau International (STTI) and the STTI ambassador to Afghanistan. Her doctoral focus is the health care of women Afghan refugees. She is a volunteer with the Georgia Refugee Health and Mental Health (GRHMH), an organization that provides health care to refugees from several countries.

Adelita Cantu, PhD, RN, is an assistant professor in the Family and Community Health Systems Department of the University of Texas Health Science Center at San Antonio. Dr. Cantu has conducted ethnographic and life history research on the initiation and sustainability of physical activity and healthy eating in older Mexican American women. She teaches population health to undergraduate students and acts as a mentor to graduate health professional students.

Nancy Capponi, MSN, RN, CEN, CCRN, is faculty in the School of Nursing undergraduate program at Clayton State University. She is currently in the EdD program (focus in Nursing Education) at the University of West Georgia. She is interested in qualitative research in the area of improving nursing education.

Mary de Chesnay, PhD, RN, PMHCNS-BC, FAAN, is professor of nursing at Kennesaw State University and secretary of the Council on Nursing and Anthropology (CONAA) of the Society for Applied Anthropology (SFAA).

She has conducted ethnographic fieldwork and participatory action research in Latin America and the Caribbean. She has taught qualitative research at all levels in the United States and abroad in the roles of faculty, head of a department of research, dean, and endowed chair.

Katrina Embrey, MSN, RN, is instructor of nursing and the undergraduate program coordinator at Armstrong Atlantic State University in Savannah, Georgia. She is currently teaching adult health nursing in both the clinical and didactic settings. She is a doctoral student at Kennesaw State University with her dissertation focus on complementary and alternative medicine.

Murray J. Fisher, PhD, RN, ICU Cert, DipAppSc, BHSc, MPHEd, is associate professor at Sydney Nursing School, University of Sydney, Australia, and nursing resident scholar at Royal Rehabilitation Centre Sydney. He has conducted theorized life histories examining men and the social embodiment of masculinities. He has taught research methods at undergraduate and postgraduate levels in Australia and abroad and has supervised several research higher degree students. He has previously held senior academic administrative roles such as director of Preregistration Programs and associate dean (Academic) at Sydney Nursing School.

Denise Haylen, RN, BN (Hons 1), CTNC, is a registered nurse and PhD student at Sydney Nursing School at the University of Sydney, Australia. She has specialized in cardiothoracic nursing and works in the Cardiothoracic Unit at St. Vincent's Hospital in Sydney. Her main research interest is in the area of illness experience using qualitative life history methods.

Tommie Nelms, PhD, RN, is professor of nursing at Kennesaw State University. She is director of the WellStar School of Nursing and coordinator of the Doctor of Nursing Science program. She has a long history of conducting and directing phenomenological research and has been a student of Heideggerian philosophy and research for many years. Her research is mainly focused on practices of mothering, caring, and family.

Jo River, RN, BN (Hons), is a lecturer and PhD candidate at the University of Sydney, Australia. Her doctoral work is a sociological study of men's health using life history method and gender relations theory. She teaches health sociology, health politics, and social determinants of health with Sydney Nursing School's masters and undergraduate programs.

Edwina Skiba-King, PhD, APN, FPMHNP-BC, PMHCNS-BC, is clinical assistant professor at Rutgers University College of Nursing in Newark, New Jersey, and treasurer of the Society of Psychiatric Advanced Practice Nurses (SPAPN). She has taught research at the graduate and undergraduate levels and served on thesis committees. As a member of the college institutional review board, she was lead reviewer for health-related proposals. A trained herbalist and energy practitioner, her clinical practice incorporates evidence-based alternative therapies.

Leslie West-Sands, PhD, APRN, FNP-BC, PMHCNS-BC, is professor, director, and dean of nursing at Jackson State Community College, Jackson, Tennessee. Her clinical practice includes mental health care in acute and community settings, as both a nurse practitioner and therapist. She has taught nursing research, theory, and evaluation at the undergraduate and graduate levels.

Foreword

A critical advantage of the life history research methodology is the ability to connect to both scientific research methodologies and those of arts and humanities. Life histories provide the flesh and blood of lived human experience to elevate statistical analysis to more than numbers. The most vibrant life histories are as compelling and riveting as great literature.

Quite commonly, life histories have been utilized as a key research methodology to understand the lives of exceptional or singular people. There seems to be no more encompassing way to understand the lives of revolutionaries, outstanding artists, great political leaders, or others who stand out within their own social group than to record their singular lives as significant individuals.

The life history approach to studying human behavior, however, extends beyond the examination of extraordinary individuals. Life histories also celebrate the genius of the grassroots and capture the scent of the everyday. Through life history accounts, we cannot only see a social group through the lens of the individual, but we can also view group social patterns as expressed by the individual's thoughts and actions. In addition, the life history experiences of a representative sample of individuals can be abstracted to apply to an understanding of a larger social group.

Life history accounts can be employed to understand variation in human thought and behavior. Utilizing the methodology can demonstrate the variant experiences among regional, religious, and ethnic groups as well as gender and socioeconomic classes. We can also come to understand how, at an individual level, internal variation within a social group can color experiences and underscore the behavioral complexity among people who may appear to be very similar. In addition, through this methodology, an individual's place within the wider social context can be examined. Life history accounts also have practical application beyond a straightforward examination of human lives. By recording life histories, catastrophic and large-scale socially significant events can be better understood by recording how individuals experience them. Knowing how people behave during such events can help prepare for their inevitable reoccurrence. In addition, life histories recorded within a troubled family or small group can highlight the family's social dynamic and make it possible to examine their problems, thus enhancing possibilities for a therapeutic outcome.

The life history methodology has proven its value in understanding lived human realities. But, as with all research methodologies, there are special considerations that accompany the use of life history. In particular, the intimate nature of life history raises certain ethical issues to be balanced with concerns about scientific rigor and accuracy.

Nursing is a field in which both research ethics and scientific validity are foremost in the design of research projects. As in all research with human subjects, nursing research projects consider the ethics of "first do no harm." Efforts to maintain scientific accuracy are to be evaluated in terms of how the research might impact the individuals whose life histories are recorded. Yet to edit a life history account by deleting all potentially sensitive material may drain the account of its vitality and immediacy. Truth is subjective and as many-sided and variant as a polygon, depending, as it does, on the perspective of the teller. Truth is also shaded by interpretation; sometimes what is left out of an account is as important as what is said. Ultimately, truth always makes someone uncomfortable.

The relationship between the one who records the life history and the one whose life history is recorded is critical. It may develop well or it may not; it may change over time. As a final note in employing the life history methodology, just as the researcher views the subject, the subject gazes back at the researcher. And both may be changed by the very intimate nature of recording a life history.

Kathleen R. Martin, PhD
Deming, New Mexico

SERIES FOREWORD

In this section, which is published in all volumes of the series, we discuss some key aspects of any qualitative design. This is basic information that might be helpful to novice researchers or those new to the designs and methods described in each chapter. The material is not meant to be rigid and prescribed because qualitative research by its nature is fluid and flexible; the reader should use any ideas that are relevant and discard any ideas that are not relevant to the specific project in mind.

Before beginning a project, it is helpful to commit to publishing it. Of course, it will be publishable because you will use every resource at hand to make sure it is of high quality and contributes to knowledge. Theses and dissertations are meaningless exercises if only the student and committee know what was learned. It is rather heart-breaking to think of all the effort that senior faculty have exerted to complete a degree and yet not to have anyone else benefit by the work. Therefore, some additional resources are included here. Appendix A for each book is a list of journals that publish qualitative research. References to the current nursing qualitative research textbooks are included so that readers may find additional material from sources cited in those chapters.

FOCUS

In qualitative research the focus is emic—what we commonly think of as "from the participant's point of view." The researcher's point of view, called "the etic view," is secondary and does not take precedence over what the participant wants to convey, because in qualitative research, the focus is on the person and his or her story. In contrast, quantitative researchers take pains to learn as much as they can about a topic and focus the research data collection on what they want to know. Cases or subjects that do not provide information about the researcher's agenda are considered outliers and are discarded or treated as aberrant data. Qualitative researchers embrace outliers and actively seek diverse points of view from participants to enrich the data. They sample for diversity within groups and welcome different perceptions even if they seek fairly homogenous samples. For example, in Leenerts and Magilvy's (2000) grounded theory study to examine self-care practices among women, they narrowed the study to low-income, White, HIV-positive women but included both lesbian and heterosexual women.

PROPOSALS

There are many excellent sources in the literature on how to write a research proposal. A couple are cited here (Annersten, 2006; Mareno, 2012; Martin, 2010; Schmelzer, 2006), and examples are found in Appendices B, C, and D. Proposals for any type of research should include basic elements about the purpose, significance, theoretical support, and methods. What is often lacking is a thorough discussion about the rationale. The rationale is needed for the overall design as well as each step in the process. Why qualitative research? Why ethnography and not phenomenology? Why go to a certain setting? Why select the participants through word of mouth? Why use one particular type of software over another to analyze data?

Other common mistakes are not doing justice to significance and failure to provide sufficient theoretical support for the approach. In qualitative research, which tends to be theory generating instead of theory testing, the author still needs to explain why the study is conducted from a particular frame of reference. For example, in some ethnographic work, there are hypotheses that are tested based on the work of prior ethnographers who studied that culture, but there is still a need to generate new theory about current phenomena within that culture from the point of view of the specific informants for the subsequent study.

Significance is underappreciated as an important component of research. Without justifying the importance of the study or the potential impact of the study, there is no case for why the study should be conducted. If a study cannot be justified, why should sponsors fund it? Why should participants agree to participate? Why should the principal investigator bother to conduct it?

COMMONALITIES IN METHODS

Interviewing Basics

One of the best resources for learning how to interview for qualitative research is by Patton (2002), and readers are referred to his book for a detailed guide to interviewing. He describes the process, issues, and challenges in a way that readers can focus their interview in a wide variety of directions that are flexible, yet rigorous. For example, in ethnography, a mix of interview methods is appropriate, ranging from unstructured interviews or informal conversation to highly structured interviews. Unless nurses are conducting mixed-design studies, most of their interviews will be semi-structured. Semi-structured interviews include a few general questions, but the interviewer is free to allow the interviewee to digress along any lines he or she wishes. It is up to the interviewer to bring the interview back to the focus of the research. This requires skill and sensitivity.

Some general guidelines apply to semi-structured interviews:

- Establish rapport.
- Ask open-ended questions. For example, the second question is much more likely to generate a meaningful response than the first in a grounded theory study of coping with cervical cancer.

  Interviewer: Were you afraid when you first heard your diagnosis of cervical cancer?

  Participant: Yes.

  Contrast the above with the following:

  Interviewer: What was your first thought when you heard your diagnosis of cervical cancer?

  Participant: I thought of my young children and how they were going to lose their mother and that they would grow up not knowing how much I loved them.

- Continuously "read" the person's reactions and adapt the approach based on response to questions. For example, in the interview about coping with the diagnosis, the participant began tearing so the interviewer appropriately gave her some time to collect herself. Maintaining silence is one of the most difficult things to learn for researchers who have been classically trained in quantitative methods. In structured interviewing, we are trained to continue despite distractions and to eliminate bias, which may involve eliminating emotion and emotional reactions to what we hear in the interview. Yet the quality of outcomes in qualitative designs may depend on the researcher–participant relationship. It is critical to be authentic and to allow the participant to be authentic.

Ethical Issues

The principles of the Belmont Commission apply to all types of research: respect, justice, beneficence. Perhaps these are even more important when interviewing people about their culture or life experiences. These are highly personal and may be painful for the person to relate, though I have found that there is a cathartic effect to participating in naturalistic research with an empathic interviewer (de Chesnay, 1991, 1993).

Rigor

Readers are referred to the classic paper on rigor in qualitative research (Sandelowski, 1986). Rather than speak of validity and reliability we use other terms, such as accuracy (Do the data represent truth as the participant sees it?) and replicability (Can the reader follow the decision trail to see why the researcher concluded as he or she did?).

DATA ANALYSIS

Analyzing data requires many decisions about how to collect data and whether to use high-tech measures such as qualitative software or old-school measures such as colored index cards. The contributors to this series provide examples of both.

Mixed designs require a balance between the assumptions of quantitative research while conducting that part and qualitative research during that phase. It can be difficult for novice researchers to keep things straight. Researchers are encouraged to learn each paradigm well and to be clear about why they use certain methods for their purposes. Each type of design can stand alone, and one should never think that qualitative research is *less than* quantitative; it is just different.

Mary de Chesnay

REFERENCES

Annersten, M. (2006). How to write a research proposal. *European Diabetes Nursing*, 3(2), 102–105.

de Chesnay, M. (1991, March 13–17). *Catharsis: Outcome of naturalistic research.* Presented to Society for Applied Anthropology, Charleston, SC.

de Chesnay, M. (1993). Workshop with Dr. Patricia Marshall of Symposium on Research Ethics in Fieldwork. Sponsored by Society for Applied Anthropology, Committee on Ethics. Memphis, March 25–29, 1992; San Antonio, Texas, March 11–14, 1993.

Leenerts, M. H., & Magilvy, K. (2000). Investing in self-care: A midrange theory of self-care grounded in the lived experience of low-income HIV-positive white women. *Advances in Nursing Science*, 22(3), 58–75.

Mareno, N. (2012). Sample qualitative research proposal: Childhood obesity in Latino families. In M. de Chesnay & B. Anderson (Eds.), *Caring for the vulnerable* (pp. 203–218). Sudbury, MA: Jones and Bartlett.

Martin, C. H. (2010). A 15-step model for writing a research proposal. *British Journal of Midwifery*, 18(12), 791–798.

Patton, M. Q. (2002). *Qualitative research and evaluation methods* (3rd ed.). Thousand Oaks, CA: Sage.

Sandelowski, M. (1986). The problem of rigor in qualitative research. *Advances in Nursing Science*, 4(3), 27–37.

Schmelzer, M. (2006). How to start a research proposal. *Gastroenterology Nursing*, 29(2), 186–188.

PREFACE

Qualitative research has evolved from a slightly disreputable beginning to wide acceptance in nursing research. Approaches that focus on the stories and perceptions of people, instead of what scientists think the world is about, have been a tradition in anthropology for a long time, and have created a body of knowledge that cannot be replicated in the lab. The richness of human experience is what qualitative research is all about. Respect for this tradition was long in coming among the scientific community. Nurses seem to have been in the forefront, though, and though many of my generation (children of the 1950s and 1960s) were classically trained in quantitative techniques, we found something lacking. Perhaps because I am a psychiatric nurse, I have been trained to listen to people tell me their stories, whether the stories are problems that nearly destroy the spirit, or uplifting accounts of how they live within their cultures, or how they cope with terrible traumas and chronic diseases. It seems logical to me that a critical part of developing new knowledge that nurses can use to help patients is to find out first what the patients themselves have to say.

In the first volume of this series, the focus is on ethnography, in many ways the grandparent of qualitative research. Subsequent volumes address grounded theory, life history, phenomenology, historical research, participatory action research, and data analysis. The volume on data analysis also includes material on focus groups and case studies, two types of research that can be used with a variety of designs, including quantitative research and mixed designs. Efforts have been made to recruit contributors from several countries to demonstrate global applicability of qualitative research.

There are many fine textbooks in nursing research that provide an overview of all the methods, but our aim here is to provide specific information to guide graduate students or experienced nurses who are novices in the designs represented in the series in conducting studies from the point of view of our constituents/patients and their families. The studies conducted by contributors provide much practical advice for beginners as well as new ideas for experienced researchers. Some authors take a formal approach, but others speak quite personally from the first person. We hope you catch their enthusiasm and have fun conducting your own studies.

Mary de Chesnay

ACKNOWLEDGMENTS

In any publishing venture, there are many people who work together to produce the final draft. The contributors kindly shared their expertise to offer advice and counsel to novices, and the reviewers ensured the quality of submissions. All of them have come up through the ranks as qualitative researchers, and their participation is critical to helping novices learn the process.

No publication is successful without great people who not only know how to do their own jobs but also how to guide authors. At Springer Publishing Company, we are indebted to Margaret Zuccarini for the idea for the series, her ongoing support, and her excellent problem-solving skills. The person who guided the editorial process and was available for numerous questions, which he patiently answered as if he had not heard them a hundred times, was Joseph Morita. Also critical to the project were the people who proofed the work, marketed the series, and transformed it from the web to hard copies, among them Chris Teja.

At Kennesaw State University, Dr. Tommie Nelms, director of the WellStar School of Nursing, was a constant source of emotional and practical support in addition to her chapter contribution to the phenomenology volume. Her administrative assistant, Mrs. Cynthia Elery, kindly assigned student assistants who completed several chores that enabled the authors to focus on the scholarship. Bradley Garner, Chadwick Brown, and Chino are our student assistants and unsung heroes of the university.

Finally, I am grateful to my cousin, Amy Dagit, whose expertise in proofreading saved many hours for some of the chapters. Any mistakes left are mine alone.

A life is not important except in the impact it has on other lives.

—Jackie Robinson, baseball player

CHAPTER ONE

OVERVIEW OF LIFE HISTORY

Mary de Chesnay

*T*elling the story of another person's life is both a fascinating venture and a privilege. When anthropologists study culture, the best teachers are often people who have spent their lives living the rituals, activities of daily living, values, and celebrations of that culture and who are willing to share their stories with outsiders. The scholarly publication of a life history can be as riveting as a thriller or mystery novel. Yet, life histories do not have to be stories of unusual people. Even the "common person's" story is of interest. Many life histories have been published in the anthropology and sociology literature, and a few in nursing are discussed in this book; yet, little is published on how to conduct a life history. In this volume, some suggestions are made for how this underused methodology might be employed to study the lives of people who, as patients, have important things to teach nurses. Some general guidelines will be provided in Chapter 3, and it is hoped that readers will adapt these for their own purposes.

OVERVIEW OF LIFE HISTORY

Philosophical Derivation

Life history is derived from ethnographic field methods in anthropology to tell the story of a key informant who is either representative of his or her culture or is articulate in discussing his or her life in order that we might better understand the culture. Life histories are collected to round out the perspective of culture from the point of view of members or to focus attention on aspects of living common to a group of people who share cultural experiences. Unlike autobiography, in which a person initiates the telling of the life story, life history is the story told by a person to a researcher. Unlike most biography, the person is a living individual whose story is framed within a cultural context rather than the historical context. Similar to life history is life story as described by Atkinson (1998). Life story is a narrative analysis of the person's life in a holistic way. The rules about conducting life story are flexible, with some researchers choosing a limited approach and some a lengthy approach similar to traditional ethnographic life histories.

To further complicate matters, life review, in which an individual works with a therapist to reflect on his or her experiences, may look like a life story or life history. The life story work that is an intervention has a rich tradition in social work and psychiatric nursing, in which it is often called reminiscence therapy. A systematic review of the literature by McKeown, Clarke, and Repper (2005) found only 14 articles using a variety of methodologies and concluded that though the literature is sparse, life story work is a sound therapeutic strategy particularly with older people.

The focus of this volume in the series on qualitative research in nursing is life history. The volume includes the process of conducting life histories and several examples, but the design is highly individualistic and needs development as a qualitative approach. Contributors present several perspectives from their own work collecting life histories and provide analysis of their experiences. Some of the chapters are reports from doctoral students who collected highly focused life histories for a class on qualitative methods. Some are from experienced researchers, and two are from doctoral students who conducted dissertation research using life history methods.

Atkinson (1998) makes the case for life stories as part science and part art. As science, the researcher follows rules of objectivity in data collection and in relaying the story as accurately as possible. As art, the researcher interprets the story within the context in which the person lived his or her life. In the life histories collected here, the authors have made an effort to respect the owners of the life history—the people telling the story—through direct quotes, while interpreting the responses in the light of the focused research questions. Chapter 2 refers the reader to original sources of a variety of life histories for a deeper understanding of the richness of the data.

Ethical Issues

Whereas the usual ethical issues of qualitative research apply to life history, there is a special twist in that the life history is the story of a person told by the person who lived it to a researcher. As such, there is a peculiar balance between privacy/confidentiality and the right to acknowledge the story. However the researcher chooses to approach the person, however long or short the interview time, it is critical to remember that the life history belongs to the person who lived the life, not to the researcher. Relaying the person's words accurately and respecting the person's right to edit the material before publication is a key difference between this method and other qualitative methods and quantitative research. In some cases, the person might want to hold the data, and it is customary to provide copies of tapes and notes as well as invite the person to edit the work before publication.

TRADITONAL LIFE HISTORY

Early ethnographers spent at least a year in the field to study cultural changes over the seasons. During this time there was adequate opportunity to get to know people who might be invited to share their life histories. Interviews were conducted over many days or months and built from establishing rapport over time to becoming involved in the person's life by being invited to family occasions. Outcomes of traditional life histories were often full-length books that captured the essence of the culture through the stories of its members. Individuals who would be willing to speak about the culture to an outsider and who would trust the ethnographer to relay the story accurately and respectfully were sought. The extended fieldwork allowed for personal relationships to develop between the ethnographer and the individuals with whom he or she interacted.

Numerous examples can be found in the anthropology literature. Only a few will be discussed here, and readers are referred to the original sources for more detail. The first published life history was by the early 19th-century anthropologist, Paul Radin, who interviewed Crashing Thunder, a Winnebago man (Radin, 1926). Radin's intent was to explain the Winnebago culture by acknowledging that cultural groups are made up of individuals, and he considered Crashing Thunder to be a man who could speak for and explain the culture through the telling of his own life story (Watson & Watson-Franke, 1985).

Later, Lurie (1966) interviewed Crashing Thunder's sister, Mountain Wolf Woman. They became close, and Mountain Wolf Woman actually lived with Lurie and her family while compiling her story, which she told over time.

Traditional life histories might be the story of one person or several within the community of interest. Grandfather Alonso, Nisa, and Black Elk are individuals with whom the ethnographers felt a personal connection and whose story they wanted to tell.

The question about whom to interview and how to approach the person is of paramount importance in life history. For without this one key informant, there is no research project. Neihardt (1932, 2008) was interested in the Messianic movement in the late 1880s that ended with the disaster at Wounded Knee and, by 1930, had developed strong relationships with the Oglala Sioux. He searched for an old Lakota medicine man who would speak with him about the spiritual significance of those days. Black Elk was one such man. He was related to the chief Crazy Horse and knew him well, and Neihardt approached him with an interpreter and the request to talk about the old days. Earlier that day, the interpreter had taken a woman to speak with Black Elk as she was writing a story about Crazy Horse, but he had politely refused. The interpreter, Neihardt, and Black Elk sat smoking together in silence for a long time, and finally Black Elk announced that he would tell his story. Whether his decision was based on gender (the male Neihardt or the female journalist) is hard to say. It might very well be that what resonated with Black Elk was the common interest in spirituality.

Other life histories collected during fieldwork are listed here so that readers interested in the traditional approach might reference them:

- *Women of Deh Koh: Lives in an Iranian Village* (Friedl, 1989)
- *Nisa: The Life and Words of a !Kung Woman* (Shostack, 1981)
- *Black Elk Speaks* (Neihardt, 1932, 2008)
- *Yaqui Women* (Kelley, 1978)
- *The Life and Times of Grandfather Alonso* (Muratorio, 1991)
- *Dona Maria's Story: Life History, Memory and Political Identity* (James, 2000)
- *Worker in the Cane: A Puerto Rican Life Story* (Mintz, 1974)
- *Becoming A Puerto Rican Espiritista: Life history of a Female Healer* (Singer & Garcia, 1989)
- *The Face of Social Suffering: Life History of a Street Drug Addict* (Singer, 2006)

FOCUSED LIFE HISTORY

Similar to the evolution of ethnography from a tradition of living in a culture for long periods of time to focusing on aspects of culture, life history has developed into focused attempts to learn about certain conditions through the experience of those who live with the condition. In nursing, we are concerned with health issues or mental health issues, but many disciplines have used life history as a research method to study experiences relevant to their practices. Hagemaster (1992) was one of the first nurses to suggest the use of life history in nursing research.

The author's work represents a focused life history or series of life histories. The first studies involved success of African Americans—what enabled successful African Americans to overcome segregation, racism, and sometimes poverty. Reported in de Chesnay (2005), this study combined semi-structured interviews, genograms, and timelines to understand the participant's story. Subsequent life histories examined what it is like to live with chronic disease (de Chesnay, Rassilyer-Bomers, Webb, & Peil, 2008 and forthcoming) and adolescent substance abuse (2012).

The work generated by de Chesnay's 2005 study demonstrates how graduate and undergraduate students can use the method to study the lives of people with disorders or conditions that interest the student. For example, one of the graduate students (Peil) had lost a close friend and was interested in how others had successfully coped with bereavement. The lead student on the substance abuse study (Walsh) had been a substance abuse counselor before entering the nursing program.

A life history of Martha Rogers was conducted by Hektor (1989) who interviewed Dr. Rogers, her friends and colleagues, and members of her family. Her focus was to document Dr. Rogers's perceptions of the life influences that led to her theory of unitary man. The article is both an excellent example of one of the few life histories conducted by nurses and the story of one of our historical figures.

SUMMARY

Life history as a method for nursing is early in development. Similar to case studies but in more depth, the life history method generates rich data that tell the story of individuals who might be ordinary in their lives but extraordinary in what they have to teach us about the culture in which they live.

REFERENCES

Atkinson, R. (1998). *The life story interview*. Thousand Oaks, CA: Sage.
de Chesnay, M. (2005). "Can't keep me down": Life histories of successful African American adults. In M. de Chesnay (Ed.), *Caring for the vulnerable*. Sudbury, MA: Jones & Bartlett.

de Chesnay, M., Rassilyer-Bomers, R., Webb, J., & Peil, R. (2008). Life histories of successful survivors of colostomy surgery, multiple sclerosis, and bereavement. In M. de Chesnay & B. Anderson (Eds.), *Caring for the vulnerable* (2nd ed.). Sudbury, MA: Jones & Bartlett.

de Chesnay, M., Walsh, L., Szekes, L., Kronawitter, V., Cox, K., Young, S., & Payne, H. (2012). Life histories of affluent adolescent substance abusers. In M. de Chesnay & B. Anderson (Eds.), *Caring for the vulnerable* (3rd ed.). Sudbury, MA: Jones & Bartlett.

Friedl, E. (1989). *The women of Deh Koh: Lives in an Iranian village.* Washington and London: Smithsonian Institution Press.

Hagemaster, J. (1992). Life history: A qualitative method of research. *Journal of Advanced Nursing, 17,* 1122–1128.

Hektor, L. (1989). Martha E. Rogers: A life history. *Nursing Science Quarterly, 2,* 63–73.

James, D. (2000). *Dona Maria's story: Life history, memory and political identity.* Durham, NC: Duke University Press.

Kelley, J. H. (1978). *Yacqui women.* Lincoln, NE: University of Nebraska Press.

Lurie, N. (1966). *Mountain Wolf Woman.* Ann Arbor: University of Michigan Press.

McKeown, J., Clarke, A., & Repper, J. (2005). Life story work in health and social care: Systematic literature review. *Journal of Advanced Nursing, 55*(2), 237–247.

Mintz, S. (1974). *Worker in the cane: A Puerto Rican life history.* New York, NY: W. W. Norton.

Muratorio, B. (1991). *The life and times of grandfather Alonso.* New Brunswick, NJ: Rutgers University Press.

Neihardt, J. (1932, 2008). *Black Elk speaks.* Albany, NY: State University of New York Press.

Radin, P. (1926). *Crashing Thunder, the autobiography of an American Indian.* NY: Appleton.

Shostack, M. (1981). *Nisa: The life and words of a !Kung Woman.* Cambridge, MA: Harvard University Press.

Singer, M. (2006). *The face of social suffering: Life history of a street drug addict.* Prospect Heights, IL: Waveland Press.

Singer, M., & Garcia, R. (1989). Becoming a Puerto Rican espiritista: Life history of a female healer. In C. Shepherd McClain (Ed.), *Women as healers* (pp. 157–185). New Brunswick, NJ: Rutgers University Press.

Watson, L. C., & Watson-Franke, M. (1985). *Interpreting life histories: An anthropological inquiry.* New Brunswick, NJ: Rutgers University Press.

CHAPTER TWO

STATE OF ART IN NURSING RESEARCH USING LIFE HISTORY

Mary de Chesnay

The second chapter in each volume in the series presents the nursing literature that uses the design that is the focus of the volume. However, life history is a design that is not much used by nurse researchers because it has been considered a method within ethnography, and nurse anthropologists currently tend to do focused ethnographies due to time constraints instead of the traditional ethnography that employs life history as part of the design. Therefore, in this chapter, most of the literature reviewed includes life histories conducted in the traditional way by anthropologists. This anthropology material is presented so that nurse researchers might become excited by the possibilities of life history as a design that has relevance and significance for the populations we study.

Several life histories conducted by nurses are presented as separate chapters in this volume. These authors have published life histories either in books such as Abrums's ethnographic work that included life histories (Abrums, 2010) or individual life histories by de Chesnay (2005, 2008, 2012) or those published in the journal literature (Cantu & Fleuriet, 2008; Hektor, 1989). In addition, two life histories that were conducted as dissertation research are presented in more detail to convey the flavor of conducting life histories as dissertations.

LIFE HISTORIES CONDUCTED BY NURSES

Martha E. Rogers by Lynn Hektor

Hektor's (1989) life history of Martha Rogers (1914–1994) was published as a journal article that documents not only the life of an extraordinary woman but also the history and culture of nursing. Most of the published work about Rogers relates to her theory and its impact on nursing, but Hektor goes beyond theory development to give us a picture of the woman who was a key figure in the history of nursing as a science. Presented chronologically, the life history is organized into four periods: childhood, years of study and work, the New York University years, and the future. At the time of publication, Rogers was still living. Interviews were conducted with Rogers, her niece, and her close friends.

The stories are presented as recollections by Rogers and paint a picture of a smart, fun-loving, and happy girl who enjoyed a close family life in the mountains of Knoxville, Tennessee.

> I remember swimming in the river, diving from my father's back, and sledding near our home in Knoxville. (p. 64)

> I remember first going to [k]indergarten. It was terribly exciting. I discovered I talked too much. I remember the teacher telling me to move away from the table. (p. 64)

In high school, she was involved in many activities of the Junior League and the Methodist Church. In college at the University of Tennessee, she considered pre-med and took a heavy science course load.

> My father was worn out buying me fertile eggs to slice up for embryos! An old farmer would always bring me fertile eggs. (p. 65)

She decided she wanted to help people and settled on a career in nursing. She completed the training program at Knoxville General Hospital and then entered George Peabody College in Nashville for a degree in public health nursing, graduating in 1937. She moved to Michigan to take a job as a public health nurse and describes her role there.

> What I did was straight public health which involved a lot of case-finding. Public health nurses planned programs, worked on committees, and were "community activists." For example, the Women's Auxiliary of the American Legion met to discuss venereal disease, and I was asked to be the speaker. (p. 66)

Rogers's years at New York University (NYU) are well-known because that is where she made her mark as a theorist, but Hektor tells the personal stories. Rogers's sense of humor is clear in her description of her first apartment.

> It was a drafty old place. The thermostat for the whole building was in my place and the woman who sublet the apartment to me put a little

cage over the thermostat and set it so the tenants couldn't change it. We put ice cubes on the top of it; this would trip the thermostat for several hours and we could warm up. (p. 68)

In discussing her influence on the NYU doctoral program, she said she had eight students in the seminar course for nurses.

I made some unilateral changes, adding statistics and later on, physics for students at all levels. That was hard for them, and I tutored students in statistics for several years. (p. 69)

Regarding how she wrote her landmark book, *An Introduction to the Theoretical Basis of Nursing* (Rogers, 1970), she described using her class notes to develop her ideas into a book.

I started with an outline I had. The thing was to get it down, to sit down with paper and pencil and write it. Then when I'd look at it, I'd ask myself—is that really stupid or what? (p. 70)

If there was anything that distinguished the division [nursing] it was the intellectual excitement, the intellectual stimulation, the sharing of ideas by everyone. (p. 71)

At the time of the interviews, Rogers had retired to spend more time with family. She reflected on her career.

Well, you know, I think people either think I'm great or I should have died a long time ago. Ten or fifteen years ago when I would give a speech, the first thing I would do would be to check out how far the windows were from the ground because really, you know, some people got very upset. (p. 72)

Patricia Morin by Linda Walline

In this dissertation, Walline (2008) was interested in the leadership qualities and formation of a nursing dean. She interviewed Patricia Morin who represented to her an ideal of women in leadership positions. When asked about her emphasis on caring, Morin explained:

Caring is more a socialization process than an actual gender (issue) . . . . I think that females have been in more caring professions—teaching, nursing, secretaries. (p. 55)

Colice Caulfield Sayer by Melissa Sherrod

Sherrod's journal article describes her study, but she does not provide the context of the study (Sherrod, 2006). Born in 1890 in New York, the daughter of a Civil War veteran, Colice Caulfield was involuntarily hospitalized in a mental hospital for 43 years by her husband. In 1914, she married Edgar Sayer with whom she had four children and enjoyed a happy family life for about 7 to 8 years. At one point, though, her husband began staying out late and "womanizing." Colice would send her children to look for him. Eventually, he told a judge that Colice was trying to kill him and asked that she be committed. Without informing her of the petition or inviting her to appear before the court, the judge complied, and she spent the next 43 years as a ward of the state of New York.

Sherrod provides the historical context of the role of women during the 1930s and also the perception of mental illness and divorce. At that time, it was not necessary to validate the person's mental status but only to verify basically that the papers of commitment were in order and that a physician had certified to the court the need for commitment. In Colice's case, the physician was only her family physician and not a psychiatrist, and the people certifying her were her husband's brother and wife. Colice described her situation:

> If I had of had a chance to fight for my sanity before I was used so inhumanely it would have been different. Certainly I said nothing insane to Dr. Sylvester. He had my papers all ready [sic] made out and no matter what I said he intended to place me here on what my enemies said. (p. 763)

Unlike life histories in which the person whose life is the subject is the main person interviewed, this study took place with Colice's children and grandchildren, a total of nine of her direct descendants. The focus of the story is the family responses to Colice's hospitalization and the loss of the mother/grandmother for a significant period of time. The author refers to the study as an edited life history, and she reviewed documents and Colice's poems and writings as well as interviewing family members. Their reactions indicate the profound disruption and lack of trust in the family.

> Edgar threw a rock into the puddle of our lives and the ripples are spreading out today. (p. 769)

> We don't ever share our experiences or feelings with other people unless they are extraordinarily close to us. I mean, my father told us that the only person we could depend on was ourselves. (p. 769)

Life Stories of African Americans by Mary de Chesnay

Arguably the most important cultural issue for African Americans has historically been overcoming racism. As a nurse, I had had many patients of color and yet felt as if I did not know them well and therefore could not be as effective a therapist as I wanted, so I conducted a study with successful African Americans to learn how they became successful. In this study, overcoming racism was universal in that all informants had stories about their experiences and how they were taught to cope with racism (de Chesnay, 2005). This study was later replicated by graduate students (de Chesnay et al., 2010) and undergraduates (de Chesnay et al., 2012) with different populations.

> I know I didn't do anything besides sit in the diner and try to eat my lunch, but when the men around me started on about being a, you know, the "n" word, I got pretty mad, but I thought about what my mama told me, and she always said they [the racist people] was ignorant and I should just pretend like I didn't hear. (p. 224)

Though the people in my study did not have much education, they all valued education and wanted to ensure it for their children:

> I was the first [in my family] to go to college and my parents were so proud of me. I have a doctoral degree now and my daddy still brags about me as if I were a little girl. . . . my brother wasn't so lucky— he would've liked to have been a doctor, but Mama got sick and [my brother] quit school to work because they didn't have insurance and Daddy didn't make much . . . ." (p. 225)

The themes of family support and church were also strong in this study, but the dominant concept that emerged from the data expressed that perseverance was the main thing that enabled these folks to thrive and not just survive. The following quote inspired the title for the study: "Can't Keep Me Down: Life Histories of Successful African Americans."

> No matter what they do to me, they can't keep me down—I always come back. (p. 226)

LIFE HISTORIES COLLECTED BY ANTHROPOLOGISTS

Life histories collected within the context of traditional fieldwork either tell the story of a singular individual or a group of people who are members of the culture of interest. Some approach the story from the point of view of the key informant and resemble an autobiography. In Radin's (1926) life history of Crashing Thunder, a Winnebago, the story is told in the first person by Crashing Thunder himself. Radin injects editorial comments to clarify aspects of the story for the reader. The following passage is an example of clarification in a footnote.

Crashing Thunder: Near the place where we lived, there were three lakes and a black-hawk's nest. Right near the tree where the nest was located, they built a lodge and our war-bundle was placed in it.

Radin: The war-bundle was the most sacred object among the Winnebago. It consisted of dried animal skins, other parts of animals, reed flutes, etc., all of which had some symbolical meaning. The various powers of these animals were supposed to give the owner the powers of those animals. The sound of the reed flutes was supposed to paralyze his enemy and make it impossible for him to walk.

(Radin, 1926, p. 17)

In the life history of Martha Rogers, Hektor spent her publishing space on a good bit of commentary by herself and the people she interviewed in addition to the direct quotes from her interviews with Rogers. In contrast, Radin allows the key informant to tell his stories in his own words with little of his own commentary.

Crashing Thunder by Paul Radin

This life history is told as a series of stories spread over his life and told by Crashing Thunder. There is a brief introduction that presents Radin's credentials for conducting the life history, and the introduction contains the most analytical statements he makes. The story itself is left to Crashing Thunder to tell. Crashing Thunder tells a candid version of his life and does not seem to edit or judge his own actions and decisions, even though he confesses to criminal activity for which he was incarcerated. He does not come across as a sociopath—far from it. His stories are presented factually from the best of his recollection, leaving the impression that he has made peace with himself in his later years. A few passages from his stories are related here to show a model of life history that is highly autobiographical without commentary by the researcher.

Childhood and Adolescence

> In the summer we always returned to Black River Falls, Wisconsin. Here all the Indians gathered after they had given their feasts. Then we picked berries . . . After a while I learned to chew tobacco and then I did not eat the berries . . . I probably used up more money in buying tobacco than would have been the value of the berries I had eaten. (p. 2)

> At this stage in my life I secretly got the desire to make myself pleasing to the opposite sex. The Indians then lived in their old-fashioned lodges. Women, however, whenever they had their menses, were placed in special huts. There the young men would go to court them at night when their parents were asleep. [My parents] did not wish me to be near menstruating women, for were I to grow up in their midst I would assuredly be weak and of little account. (p. 16)

The stories are not told as a history of the Winnebago people, yet it is clear from Crashing Thunder's experiences that the white settlement of the West greatly influenced his life. He describes a long history of alcoholism, living off the annuities given to the various women he "married," and stealing instead of working. His stories of childhood depict the hunting culture of his father and older brothers, while his young adult life straddled the two worlds of traditional life and white domination. One example is the western shows he participated in as a dancer.

> Eventually the show was over and we all went to our homes. We had to go across Lake Michigan. It was very stormy and we all got sick. Then [my friend] took out some whiskey which he was carrying in a flask and we drank all night. (p. 131)

At one point, his parents joined a group of Indians that used peyote, a hallucinogenic plant found in Mexico and the American southwest that has been treated as a divine herb for centuries by indigenous people and adopted by the Native American Church for their rituals (Stewart, 1987). He was asked to join them but resisted at first because he believed that the peyote was one of the "four spirits from below," meaning bad and leading people to behave badly.

> Those who use the peyote claim that when they die, they will only be going on a long journey. But that is not the truth, for when they eat peyote, they destroy their souls, and death to them will mean complete extermination. (pp. 169–170)

Despite his conviction, he later participated in a peyote ceremony and claimed to be cured, though he does not specify the disease. His wife suffered as well and became very sick, and he urged her to take the peyote. She ate it and recovered.

> I painted her face and took her gourd and began singing to her very much. Then I stopped. "You are right," she said, "for now I am well." From that day she has been well. Now she is very happy. (p. 182)

How can nurse researchers use Radin's form of life history to tell the story of a person of interest to nursing? Radin found a person representative of the culture he wanted to study in a detailed way, and his interviews with Crashing Thunder took place over the course of several seasons when he would travel to visit the reservation. Hektor had access to Martha Rogers, a person representative of nursing culture. These people can be considered of special interest because of the time they lived in and their accomplishments, but anyone's life is worth telling because we all have something to learn from each other.

Mama Lola by Karen M. Brown

A third example of style in conducting life history research is Brown's work with Mama Lola, whose given name is Alourdes, a Haitian immigrant to New York City. Brown (1991) describes her evolution from a researcher to friend to member of Alourdes' extended family. The book was first described as a postmodern feminist ethnography, a label Brown seems reluctant to accept. Regardless of labeling, the book shows extensive participant observation over years of interaction with Alourdes and the deep affection with which she and Alourdes treated each other.

In contrast to Radin's work with Crashing Thunder, Brown actively participated in many of the family gatherings and vodou ceremonies that she described in the book. She was actually initiated into the religion and traveled to Haiti with Alourdes to visit family there.

SUMMARY

Though life histories in nursing are relatively rare, the technique is used and demonstrates the richness of data when the data are generated by the person who owns the story. There really is no substitute for having skilled and empathic interviewers elicit the stories directly from the people who lived them. As a qualitative method, life history can tell us much about how patients and their families interpret their health conditions, make decisions, and solve the many problems they experience, whether healthy or ill. When viewed within the context of the culture of the patient and community, life stories can lead to new solutions that health care providers can use to develop better interventions and policies.

REFERENCES

Abrums, M. E. (2010). *Moving the rock: Poverty and faith in a black storefront church.* Lanham, MD: Alta Mira Press.

Brown, K. M. (1991). *Mama Lola: A vodou priestess in Brooklyn.* Berkeley, CA: University of California Press.

Cantu, A. G., & Fleuriet, K. J. (2008). Sociocultural context of physical activity in older Mexican American women. *Hispanic Health Care International, 6,* 1–20.

de Chesnay, M. (2005). "Can't keep me down": Life histories of successful African American adults. In M. de Chesnay (Ed.), *Caring for the vulnerable.* Sudbury, MA: Jones & Bartlett.

de Chesnay, M., Rassilyer-Bomers, R., Webb, J., & Peil, R. (2008). Life histories of successful survivors of colostomy surgery, multiple sclerosis, and bereavement. In M. de Chesnay & B. Anderson (Eds.), *Caring for the vulnerable* (2nd ed.). Sudbury, MA: Jones & Bartlett.

de Chesnay, M., Walsh, L., Szekes, L., Kronawitter, V., Cox. K., Young, S., & Payne, H. (2012). In M. de Chesnay & B. Anderson (Eds.), *Caring for the vulnerable* (3rd ed.). Sudbury, MA: Jones & Bartlett.

Hektor, L. (1989). Martha E. Rogers: A life history. *Nursing Science Quarterly, 2,* 63–73.

Radin, P. (1926). *Crashing Thunder: An autobiography of an American Indian.* Ann Arbor, MI: University of Michigan Press.

Rogers, M. E. (1970). *An introduction to the theoretical basis of nursing.* New York, NY: F.A. Davis.

Sherrod, M. (2006). Colice's story and the effects of generational loss. *Western Journal of Nursing Research, 28,* 754–777.

Stewart, O. (1987). *Peyote religion: A history.* Norman, OK: University of Oklahoma Press.

Walline, L. K. (2008). *The life of Patricia Morin: A nursing dean.* Open Access Theses and Dissertations from the College of Education and Human sciences, University of Nebraska, Lincoln. Paper 25. http://digitalcommons.unl.edu/cehsdiss/25

CHAPTER THREE

COLLECTING LIFE HISTORIES

Mary de Chesnay and Murray J. Fisher

*L*ife histories give voice to the ordinary members of a culture as they cope on a daily basis with the joys and challenges of life. Each person has a story to tell, and one can learn as much from an ordinary person as from a celebrity or community leader. This chapter provides a guide to conducting a life history from conceptualization to dissemination.

The life history method aims to document a person's life or a significant part of life as narrative, through the telling and recording of one's life (Plummer, 2001). The life story (biography) is not the life experience but a representation of it and is a way of organizing the experience and fashioning or verifying identity (Atkinson, 1998). The life story is a constructed account, a representation of the life as lived, which is interpreted and reconstructed in a historical moment by the informant (Denzin, 1989). Despite the life story being a reconstruction, the personal narrative (life story) is a most helpful way to gain a perspective on, and understanding of, the experiences of individuals.

Life history is used to explain an individual's understanding of social events, movements, and political causes, that is, how individual members of groups or institutions see certain events and how they experience and interpret those events. The life history can help the researcher define a person's place in the social order of things, the processes used, and social structures that influence social relations.

Plummer (2001), in his book *Documents of Life 2*, outlines the distinctions between different kinds of life stories: the long and the short; the comprehensive, the topical, and the edited; and the naturalistic, researched, and reflexive. Unlike the comprehensive life story, the topical life story, according to Plummer (2001), does not aim to grasp the totality of the informant's life but rather examines a highly focused area of life. These life stories are edited and woven together to create a map of sociological meaning. The life stories produced are not naturalistic; they did not naturally occur but were researched to bring into being sociological life histories that otherwise would not have been evident in everyday life.

CONCEPTUALIZATION

As it is unlikely that nurses will be conducting traditional fieldwork to gather life histories because of the extensive periods of time involved, we will describe the process for collecting focused life histories by researchers whose only purpose is to document the story of the participant and not to frame this life history within a broader ethnography. Participant observation and other fieldwork may or may not be involved depending on the degree to which the participant may invite the researcher into his or her life. For example, during the course of interviews, the person living with a chronic disease may be hospitalized and the researcher would visit the hospital. The purpose of the visit is not to conduct a formal interview but to maintain the caring attitude one has established with the participant.

Statement of the Problem

Deciding what to study and framing the research question can be the hardest parts of a research study. In life history, though, the researcher is usually intrigued by the lives or culture of a group and wishes to learn more about the culture as seen through the eyes of those who live there. Traditional life histories were collected with people thought to be excellent and articulate representations of their culture, most frequently meaning older men. Gradually ethnographers discovered other members of the culture and realized that even women and young people have something to offer.

Literature Review

How much literature to review before beginning the study is somewhat controversial. Some believe that prior review of the complete literature on a topic prejudices the researcher to the point where he or she cannot hear what the participant says. We favor enough literature review to determine whether the study needs to be done. This would involve collecting background on the problem and the setting but not so much on the condition of interest (e.g., bereavement, chronic disease). Authors of the various chapters in each volume will have conflicting views on the extent of the literature review, and the decision lies ultimately with the researcher (and the doctoral committee).

Significance of the Study

One of the most important aspects of conducting research is to justify the study. The investigator's and participants' time and effort, and possibly a sponsor's money, need to be spent to generate knowledge—either for its own sake to preserve the culture of isolated peoples or to lay the groundwork for interventions that will help people. Trivial questions waste time and energy and can be viewed as insulting by the participants. We cannot stress enough that the study needs to be justified. Significance is much more than a simple claim, "This study is significant to nursing." Significance involves stating how the study is significant, "The results from this study on how African American adults successfully overcome racism will help the researcher to develop interventions to enhance skills in African American children and support systems in African American families to prevent and mitigate the effects of racism."

METHODOLOGICAL PHASE

Hagemaster (1992) was one of the first nurse researchers to publish a guide to collecting life histories. She proposed a six-step process from learning about qualitative research techniques in general to proceeding through field interviews, ongoing analysis, and literature reviews. This was a short journal article and provided the broad strokes but did not discuss the myriad issues and challenges likely to arise when conducting the research.

Design

The type of life history to be collected depends on the resources of the researcher, the cultural phenomenon of interest, the research question, and the ability to recruit appropriate participants. In this volume, we treat life history as a sociocultural methodology and leave oral history to the volume on historical research and life review to the one on clinical literature. Therefore, we stress the key informant's cultural context and social influences rather than chronological events or memories of a pivotal event. For example, oral histories would be more important when the researcher is interested in memories of people who were present during a specific time.

- Where were you when Kennedy was shot? What did you do? How did you feel?
- What were your experiences as a military nurse in Europe during World War II?
- What was it like to practice as a nurse midwife in South Africa under apartheid?
- What was it like to be a slave in colonial America? (oral histories of former slaves were collected by the Works Progress Administration during the Great Depression).
- What health care was provided during the great flu epidemic of 1919?

Life review stories are not research but rather a clinical tool for helping people synthesize their experiences. This technique is sometimes called reminiscence therapy and can be quite useful with the elderly or with terminally ill patients.

Sampling

Recruiting the key informant can be done by personal contacts through work or community contacts. The major task is to identify a key informant or participant whose life involves the culture or condition of interest. Several students who conducted life histories under the guidance of the authors identified their participants by personal knowledge of their condition. Becca, a graduate student, had experienced a personal bereavement and sought advice from a woman who had gone through a similar loss. Renee and Jessica, also nurse practitioners and graduate students, collected life histories of former patients who had undergone colostomy (Renee) or had multiple sclerosis (Jessica) after the patients had recovered (de Chesnay, Rassilyer-Bomers, Webb, & Peil, 2008). Lisa and her colleagues had worked with substance abusers and had former patients who were affluent adolescents recovering from alcohol and drug addictions (de Chesnay et al., 2012).

Purposive Sampling With Snowballing

For qualitative research, the sampling method is usually purposive, meaning that one identifies the types of participants one needs and then looks for a few people who fit the criteria among colleagues, acquaintances, fieldwork contacts, or formal agencies. In the case of life history, it may only be necessary to find one key informant (Muratorio, 1991; Neihardt, 2008; Shostack, 1981).

Often, groups of life histories are collected (Abrums, 2010; de Chesnay. 2005; Kelley, 1978). Once the initial participants are interviewed, if more than one is desired, the technique called snowballing (or sometimes called network sampling) is often used. This means one asks the first people interviewed to recommend others who might be contacted. For example, in the initial study on successful African Americans, most of the 22 participants were identified through snowballing—referrals from previous interviewees. In one case, a busy judge refused to be interviewed until he heard that his childhood minister had suggested him. His whole demeanor changed, and he not only made time immediately but spent much more time in sessions than needed. He made it clear that the high degree of respect he had for the minister was the reason he agreed to help.

Quantitative research aims to test representative samples of the population and makes inferences about the population, thus requiring a probability (random) sample. In quantitative research, the sampling method used when one cannot obtain the best (random) sample is called a convenience sampling. We object to this term for qualitative research because it does not capture the effort that goes into purposive sampling and snowballing. The connotation in the term sample of convenience makes it sound as if the researcher is settling for something less than adequate. In reality, purposive sampling is organized, deliberate, and precise. Unlike quantitative research, life history research does not require a random sample, as the life story only represents the participant who told the story. Like most qualitative research methods, the aim of life history research is not to make generalizations or inferences about the population but rather find similarities and differences across participants.

Snowballing is also purposive in that the early participants, once interviewed, know what the researcher is after and may know people with similar circumstances. In a study of men in nursing (Fisher, 2009), the sampling strategy combined snowball sampling with quota sampling. The researcher believed it was important to ensure that men from all areas of nursing practice were included, so the sampling strategy included selecting four men in each of five broad categories of nursing: medical–surgical; critical care; pediatrics, gynecology, and midwifery (obstetric nursing); aged care and palliative care; and mental health. Snowball sampling was used when male nurses were asked if they knew other men working in the same field of nursing.

Gender

Gender ideology and standards of appropriate behavior between men and women in many societies are culturally determined. This can cause complications when the researcher and participants are of different sex. Women researchers may have to learn how to deal with sexual advances from male members of the society and that, if they accept such advances, they are not likely to be taken seriously by the women in that community, who may be threatened by their presence. Appropriate standards for women may also differ based on marital status and whether the researcher has children, as participants might view married women with children as having higher status in their own society, whether it is true or not. For example, the Yaqui women interviewed by Kelley (1978) clearly would have related their stories to a male researcher in a different way than they did to Kelley, a married woman with children.

This is not to say that men cannot interview women nor women cannot interview men. As Watson and Watson-Frank (1985) point out, the effectiveness of the interviewer depends on the ability to convey sensitivity, interest, and respect. Linderman's (1972) work with Pretty Shield, a Crow medicine woman illustrates that mutual respect trumps gender. This is further illustrated in the sensitive study on male suicide by Jo River and Murray Fisher in this volume and the study of women's recovery from acute coronary syndrome (Gallagher, Marshall, & Fisher 2010) in which many interviews were conducted by a male.

Institutional Review Board

The institutional review boards (IRBs; also known as human research ethics committees in some countries)—created after the Belmont Report to the U.S. Congress mandated that they be set up to protect the rights of human subjects—were dominated in many institutions by the "hard" sciences in the early days. However, in the last 10 years, concerted efforts have been made to include members from the social sciences who are more familiar with qualitative methods. Formerly it was difficult to obtain approval for a qualitative study, but now most institutions are more sophisticated and able to review qualitative studies as easily as quantitative research. As nurses obtained doctoral degrees, they became members of IRBs and have also had an influence on the approval process.

Two issues with IRBs might continue to be problems. The nature of obtaining consent in developing countries or with populations deeply suspicious of being asked to sign consent forms necessitates finding alternative ways of documenting consent. One solution is to conduct verbal consent on audiotape, easily done if the interviews are to be taped. The other has to do with use of pseudonyms. Researchers might be committed to confidentiality, but failure to use the participant's real name might be insulting to some people. For example, in a study by de Chesnay (1986) on Jamaican family structure, one key informant insisted that his real name be used because he carried his father's name and was proud of his father. We compromised and used his middle name.

Universals for documenting the protection of human subjects are assurance of confidentiality and providing a calm atmosphere without coercion. Assuring anonymity is not possible because the researcher knows the participant, but every effort must be made to conduct the interviews in a respectful manner and to protect the raw data. This also involves protecting the privacy of associated persons or agencies that could identify the participants.

Whereas the use of pseudonyms aims to de-identify participants, caution needs to be undertaken in the presentation of people's lives to ensure that other features of an individual's life are also sufficiently de-identified. This may also be dependent on the population that is being studied. For example, in a study of male nurses in Australia (Fisher, 2009), caution was taken to ensure that locations of individuals and position titles were sufficiently altered to maintain confidentiality. Whereas there were over 5,000 male nurses registered in New South Wales, Australia, the employment position of some of the participants made them easily identifiable. In the chapter by Haylen and Fisher, which presents a study of women's experiences of a rare disease, the authors highlight the difficulty in maintaining participant confidentiality for participants drawn from a small population.

Incentives

Incentives should be used carefully because it is important to avoid undue pressure on the participant. Kelley (1978) discussed the gifts she gave and the favors she did for members of the community when she collected life histories of Yaqui women. Because she defined incentives as gifts, she reported that the women reciprocated by giving her gifts such as handmade clothing and food in return. They did not define their participation in the study as reciprocation. She would often take women on excursions to the beach or shopping in her car so that they did not have to walk or take the unreliable local transportation. These small services enabled her to reciprocate in other ways that were respectful to the women. In general, most people are willing to share their personal story without incentives and are appreciative of the time taken to listen to and the interest shown in their life story.

Instrumentation

Life history research usually includes interviews over time and review of any documents or artifacts of relevance. However, the primary instrument of research is the interviewer, because without the ability to establish rapport and trust, the interviews are likely to be meaningless.

Researcher as Instrument

In qualitative research, the investigator is the primary instrument, for it is in the skill of the interviewer that the best data are obtained. Nurses may find it easier to establish rapport because people may have more experience talking to nurses rather than other strangers. Using simple interview/communication skills can assist with establishing rapport with participants. Taking the time to establish a relationship with the participants is key to success at interviewing. There are many sources on how to interview, and one highly recommended source is by Patton (2002).

Setting

Life history interviews and participant observations can be conducted in any setting. It is important that life history interviews are conducted in a comfortable and quiet location where there are minimal interruptions. Life history observations and interviews are often conducted at the participant's residential address, as it is convenient for the participant and reduces the travel burden. This also allows the researcher to take field notes regarding the participant's interactions with his or her own environment. However, conducting interviews in participants' homes may create safety risks and limits your control of interruptions. If interviews are to be conducted in the participant's environment (home or workplace, etc.), then a safety risk procedure should be developed. For this reason, it is often advisable to conduct interviews in a neutral but mutually agreed location. A test recording at the interview location should be conducted prior to commencing the interview to ensure there is minimal background noise or recording distortions.

Rigor

In qualitative research, rather than speak of validity and reliability, we use accuracy, confirmability, replicability, and transferability. In life history, no two researchers will elicit the same life story from a participant. Similarly, if you were to elicit a participant's life story on two occasions, you will never get the same life story. The telling of a life story is dependent on memory, a memory shaped by culture, religion, and sociopolitical forces. As a health researcher doing life history you are interested in the subjective story of the participants, their interpretations, and meaning of key events. Stories will be value laden and value driven, and it is the dialectical relationship between researcher and participant that co-creates the life story. It is the subjective reality of the story at the time of the telling that is the truth (Denzin, 1989). Unlike in other qualitative research, it is not common practice in life history to give transcripts of interviews back to participants for confirmation, as the story told at a particular time is taken to be the truth.

The researcher must decide whether the accuracy of the history of events is important in the interpretation of the life history. If accuracy is important, then data sources other than participant interviews may be used to confirm participant stories. Diaries, medical records, or other documents can be used as data to inform and confirm the history of events. The chapter by Haylen reports that, in her study of women with a rare life-threatening illness, she utilized participant medical records to confirm the accuracy of events and to provide data to shape the biographical account of each participant.

On the other hand, it may not be necessary to confirm details, particularly if the philosophical approach is to relate the story as told by the narrator. In this sense, the interest is in how the person tells the story rather than the facts of the story. For example, in the life history of successful African American adults (de Chesnay, 2005), one man told me he had witnessed the lynching of a Black man he called his uncle. He placed the lynching in the early 20th century in rural South Carolina when he was a small boy. The way he remembered the story was that the man had been seen "courting a White girl." The family story was that the man and young woman had been childhood friends and were simply talking about old times. Although it would be good to be able to check the historical record of the lynching, it is highly unlikely that the official record would be truthful because the public record would have been written by a segregationist law enforcement office and a biased press. What is significant in this story is the effect it had on the boy who grew up believing it and adapted his own behavior toward White women accordingly.

Procedures for Data Collection

The way and the order in which data are collected are highly individual and depend on what data the interviewer needs in order to tell the story. For some life histories, such as the one for Martha Rogers, other people such as family members and colleagues are interviewed (Hektor, 1989). In the studies by de Chesnay (2005, 2008, 2012), genograms and timelines were collected. In some traditional life histories (Brown, 1991; Radin, 1926), data are collected over years of visits to the person.

Data Analysis

Data analysis in life history research is not well discussed in the published works and varies depending on the purpose of the research. Life histories can be reported in many ways ranging from an autobiographical account with little interpretation from the researcher through to sophisticated theorized life histories. Data analysis for life history is often in the form of narrative analysis. Described briefly here, narrative analysis is simply a way of examining the linguistic elements of a story. Readers are referred to a subsequent volume of this series, titled *Data Analysis,* for a more thorough treatment of discourse analysis, narrative analysis, and content analysis.

Theoretical life histories may require alternate analytical procedures. For example, in a study that examined the lived experience of men who are or have been obese using a gender relations approach, Fisher and Chilko (2012) investigated the impact of obesity on identity, social practice, and gender relations in order to discover why individuals are successful (or not) in changing their lifestyles and behaviors. Life history methodology was used to collect personal narratives from obese men to explain their understanding of social events, movements, and political causes, and to explain how individual members of groups or institutions see, experience, and interpret those events. Each life story underwent a structural analysis of the narrative in which the gender relations approach and the gender substructures (Connell, 1995, 2000, 2002) were applied to the data to inform key patterns of gender. Data analysis consisted of the identification of patterns of social response and the identification of themes. This approach to analysis is consistent with other life history research on gender such as Connell's classic study of masculinities (Connell, 1995), Fisher's study of male nurses (Fisher, 2009), and River's study on male suicide (see Chapter 7 in this volume).

Timelines for life history are as long as it takes to complete the data collection. The study design, data type, and recruitment strategy can impact the study's timeline. Some studies require multiple interviews for each participant, whereas other studies require one interview. If the life history is highly focused, fewer interviews are needed. If the life history is more like an autobiography, the data collection can extend over several years. If data are collected from patients from multiple sites, ethical approval may be required from each site and may delay the commencement of data collection.

Writing the report requires a number of decisions: what to include, how much to include, when to develop several papers from one study, and whether to publish as a book or a journal article. Whichever form is chosen, it is important to disseminate the story. It is also important to follow up with the participant or key informant. The person has told the story of his or her life for a purpose, not to have it forgotten by a researcher too shy to submit the work to external review.

REFERENCES

Abrums, M. (2010). *Moving the rock: Poverty and faith in a black storefront church.* Lanham, MD: Alta Mira Press.

Atkinson, R. (1998). *The life story interview.* Thousand Oaks, CA: Sage.

Brown, K. M. (1991). *Mama Lola: A Vodou priestess in Brooklyn.* Berkeley, CA: University of California Press.

Connell, R. W. (1995). *Masculinities.* Cambridge: Polity Press; Sydney: Allen & Unwin; Berkeley, CA: University of California Press.

Connell, R. W. (2000). *The men and the boys.* Sydney: Allen & Unwin; Cambridge: Polity Press; Berkeley: CA, University of California Press.

Connell, R. W. (2002). *Gender.* Cambridge, MA, Polity Press; Malden: MA, Blackwell.

de Chesnay, M. (1986). Jamaican family structure: The paradox of normalcy. *Family Process, 25,* 293–300.

de Chesnay, M. (2005). "Can't keep me down": Life histories of successful African American adults. In M. de Chesnay (Ed.), *Caring for the vulnerable.* Sudbury, MA: Jones & Bartlett.

de Chesnay, M., Rassilyer-Bomers, R., Webb, J., & Peil, R. (2008). Life histories of successful survivors of colostomy surgery, multiple sclerosis, and bereavement. In M. de Chesnay & B. Anderson (Eds.), *Caring for the vulnerable* (2nd ed.). Sudbury, MA: Jones & Bartlett.

de Chesnay, M., Walsh, L., Szekes, L., Kronawitter, V., Cox. K., Young, S., & Payne, H. (2012). In M. de Chesnay & B. Anderson (Eds.), *Caring for the vulnerable* (3rd ed.). Sudbury, MA: Jones & Bartlett.

Denzin, N. K., (1989). *Interpretive biography—Qualitative research methods series 17.* London, UK: Sage.

Fisher, M. (2009). "Being a Chameleon": Labour processes of male nurses performing bodywork. *Journal of Advanced Nursing, 65*(12), 2668–2677.

Fisher, M., & Chilko, N. (2012). Gender and obesity. In Louise A. Baur, Stephen M. Twigg, Roger S. Magnusson (Eds.), *A modern epidemic: Expert perspectives on obesity and diabetes* (pp. 107–119). Sydney, Australia: Sydney University Press.

Gallagher, R., Marshall, A., & Fisher, M. (2010). Symptoms and treatment-seeking responses in women experiencing acute coronary syndrome for the first time. *Heart and Lung: the Journal of Acute and Critical Care, 39*(6), 477–484.

Hagemaster, J. (1992). Life history: A qualitative method of research. *Journal of Advanced Nursing, 17*, 1122–1128.

Hektor, L. (1989). Martha E. Rogers: A life history. *Nursing Science Quarterly, 2*, 63–73.

Kelley, J. H. (1978). *Yaqui women*. Lincoln, NE: University of Nebraska Press.

Linderman, F. B. (1972). *Pretty Shield: Medicine woman of the Crow*. New York, NY: John Day.

Muratorio, B. (1991). *The life and times of grandfather Alonzo*. New Brunswick, NJ: Rutgers University Press.

Neihardt, J. G. (2008). *Black Elk speaks*. Albany, NY: State University of New York Press.

Patton, M. Q. (2002). *Qualitative research and evaluation methods*. Thousand Oaks, CA: Sage.

Plummer, K. (2001). *Documents of life: An invitation to a critical humanism*. London, UK: Sage.

Radin. P. (1926). *Crashing thunder: An autobiography of an American Indian*. Ann Arbor, MI: University of Michigan Press.

Shostack, M. (1981). *Nisa: The life and words of a !Kung woman*. Cambridge, MA: Harvard University Press.

Watson, L., & Watson-Frank, M. (1985). *Interpreting life histories*. New Brunswick, NJ: Rutgers University Press.

CHAPTER FOUR

EMBRACING THE UGLY CHILD WITHIN: LIFE HISTORY OF AN INCEST SURVIVOR

Leslie West-Sands

This study was conducted as part of doctoral degree requirements, and the following comments are offered to help provide a frame of reference for and insight into the experience of conducting this study. Prior to conducting this study, I had spent a year studying the purposes and varying processes of theory-generating and theory-testing research within the context of developing disciplined knowledge. At the time, published research was almost exclusively quantitative and thus widely considered superior to qualitative research. Skill in quantitative data analysis was a core competency of the graduate curriculum, and as a student, I was eager to use power analysis to prescribe sufficient sample size. I coveted my classmate's purchase of the latest statistical analysis software, which enabled her to quickly answer the most important question of all: Is the finding statistically significant? (Ironically, I didn't even own a computer, yet I still wanted the software, for use with a mainframe maybe?) Both the master's and doctoral programs I had chosen touted long-standing, established traditions of quality research, and I quickly became a loyal consumer of published research.

My initial exposure to qualitative research came during my first term of doctoral study, and I recall my response as fairly dismissive; I thought it could possibly support descriptive-level work of a basic nature, but the lack of robust measurement, controls, and generalizable findings did not equate to what I knew to be "true" research. Or so I thought. That's the thing about paradigms: Once adopted, allegiance limits objectivity.

It was the practice of the doctoral program I attended to host symposia for upper-level students, who were completing coursework and preparing to begin dissertation research, to present their preliminary dissertation research proposals for discussion and to receive feedback from faculty members outside of their dissertation committee. While listening to the proposed research of the senior-level students, I quickly appreciated how deeply invested they had become in their chosen topics and how genuinely they desired to create some meaningful contribution to the discipline's knowledge base. I remember feeling perplexed but did not yet understand why. I understood the research plans I had heard, but the experience of hearing multiple proposals, one after the other, each of which planned isolation and quantification of specific variables with control of foreseeable influence and error, and then asserting the findings obtained to be generalizable for developing knowledge of complex, interrelated phenomena for use in developing discipline-specific interventions for the benefit of humans (who are complex systems, inherently interrelated with both others and their environment) struck me as both odd and confusing. A disconnect between the planned methods of investigation, measurements, and data analysis suddenly seemed evident with the planned use of the data. I had become aware of conceptual inconsistencies and began experiencing cognitive dissonance.

If there was anything I felt more certain about than the power of statistical measures, it would be the utility of systems theory, which had become my favored framework for processing new information and experiences. Although I did not realize it at the time, my attempts to frame this experience from a systems theory perspective only served to fuel the cognitive dissonance experienced. I recall questioning if I had chosen the wrong discipline, but I continued to follow the doctoral curriculum in the hope that my confusion would be resolved. Each term, I delved deeper into theoretical and research literature and began to wonder if there could be more to qualitative research than I had assumed. Yet I found few published qualitative nursing research studies (outside of a quarterly journal dedicated to qualitative nursing research), but once I began looking for it, I found qualitative research to be plentiful in the publications outside of nursing, in anthropology, sociology, and even psychology.

The following year, I again attended the research proposal presentations of classmates and finally realized the source of my confusion: I had grown to doubt the universal utility of what I knew to be research because I had limited my definition of research to the reductionist paradigm of quantitative design. After reading and analyzing qualitative studies, my allegiance began to transition from valuing the precision of isolating and quantifying, controlling and generalizing to appreciating multiple methods of assessment and measurement of phenomena, within the context of their interrelated functioning.

At that time, only a few of the graduate faculty members were versed in qualitative methods, but those who were provided invaluable guidance and encouragement. One of them directed me to explore literature and mentors from other disciplines, which proved pivotal to my learning. Exposure to the acceptance and utility of qualitative research designs by other disciplines led me to pursue formalized training, via interprofessional graduate coursework, in qualitative research design and methods. This experiential course included the design and implementation of eight, small-scale qualitative studies, along with data analysis appropriate to each design, which provided invaluable experience to practice a range of qualitative techniques. The experiences gained in this course also solidified my suspicions regarding the utility of the reductionist paradigm for human studies, a thought I had never even entertained prior to exploring qualitative research. The process of learning "how" to conduct research had indoctrinated my understanding into a singular perspective. By nature paradigms are limiting, and gaining appreciation for the utility of both qualitative and quantitative research has been pivotal for both my education and practice. With the guidance of several graduate faculty members from the disciplines of nursing, education, and sociology, a study that sought a deep understanding of the phenomena of interest from a single, exemplar subject took shape; at that time, this method was untried and unfamiliar to many.

While planning for the study data collection, the construct of incest was thoroughly analyzed. A concept analysis was not prescribed prior to conducting a life history, as it may have tainted my perceptions and interpretation of the information provided by the respondent. However, because a conceptual analysis and review of theoretical and research literature were required components of dissertation proposals, these were completed according to guidelines.

The use of a single subject, albeit an exemplar, was foreign to my classmates, and one of them asked, "Why just the one?" during the discussion portion of my doctoral proposal presentation. I thought it was an obvious question and eagerly responded to share my new-found knowledge of the tenets of naturalistic inquiry as well as the life history method; several classmates expressed new interest in learning more about the sampling structures of qualitative designs.

A background in therapeutic interviewing, and experience in observing and interpreting communications, is recommended for those planning investigations using "self" as an instrument of measurement. More often than not, the context, body language, and tone of communication(s) relay more meaning than semantics. Whether pursuing an unobtrusive measure or life history, observation and interviewing skills are essential to the collection and interpretation of data. In this particular study, many of the skills acquired during a year of training as a clinical therapist were used to facilitate disclosure, seek clarification, and interpret data from the emic view. Although clinical training is not a prerequisite, the saying "dirt in, dirt out" is as applicable to the components of qualitative studies as it is to quantitative research. Deficient therapeutic skills will likely limit sensitivity to data and the collection process and subsequent data interpretation and utility. The use of specific, even brief, guided experiential exercises to practice, develop, and refine interviewing, communication interpretation, and relationship termination skills is highly recommended for those interested in pursuing the life history method.

Once I cleared the hurdles of gaining approval of the graduate school and the institutional review board, I was eager to begin data collection, but I quickly realized that the attainment of my academic goals was not going to be the primary outcome of this experience. The experience of listening with undivided attention and being fully present, physically, emotionally, and cognitively, while the respondent talked, at first, in a nondirected fashion, and later in detail, forever changed my thoughts, feelings, and perspective about the constructs of incest and survival of sexual victimization. Qualitative techniques require investments of time; life histories, in particular, require significant personal energy and time, which will very likely change both the researcher and respondent. Even though my prior training as a therapist had taught me techniques of controlling communication and to separate personal emotions from the phenomena being investigated, I recall feeling angry at times during data collection and being tearful when terminating the relationship with the respondent. Prepare to be personally affected by the life history method, as it requires both the researcher and respondent to develop trust and share themselves with each other in ways rarely found in quantitative studies.

The time required for the data interpretation phase exceeded that of the data collection phase, which surprised me. I remember thinking how time efficient statistics had been with my master's thesis and at one point wished for a correlate to the step-wise multiple regression. The respondent was articulate and freely verbal, producing many hours of audiotape for transcription.

In the noting relations phase of this study, I found a few singular data units that were unrelated to any of the categories generated from the data. In an effort to improve consistency, I chose to repeat the data categorization steps, so I set the data units aside for a few days and worked on other projects. I purposefully took a break from the data in the hope of obtaining a more consistent categorization. When I returned to the data, I reread each of the data units and again sorted them into content categories. This time there were only a few cards that stood alone. Clarification was sought from the respondent by asking for more information about the piece of data on these cards to help me connect the data to a category. By asking the respondent to "tell me more about . . .," I was able to gain greater insight into the meaning she attributed to the data; this clarified the categorization. The respondent also checked the data categories and provided feedback regarding the internal consistency, or lack thereof, of the data clusters.

Attempts to provide thick description were also time consuming, as I struggled to find words that would accurately and adequately capture the meaning and emotion relayed by the respondent. In the original dissertation, 319 direct quotes were used to provide thick description and conceptual clarity of the phenomena of interest.

Lastly, the experience of conducting research with a single subject taught me about unintentional bias among colleagues and the importance of remaining open to views and methods that differ from our own. Granted, from a quantitative perspective, data generated from a single subject are considered meaningless for generating reputable and generalizable results. However, in qualitative designs, it is the depth of data collection and time of immersion in the respondent's experience that supports accurate data collection and interpretation. Those familiar with statistical analysis programs will find that the time required for analysis of qualitative data far exceeds that needed for even the most complex statistical analyses. The analogy that comes to mind is it is as different as mowing a yard with a self-propelled mower and hand-cutting the grass (with a pair of nail clippers) after careful examination of each blade of grass and its relationship to other blades in the lawn.

It is my hope that this chapter will be helpful without discouraging students interested in pursuing the life history method. I found it to be the most rewarding research experience I could have imagined and encourage you to invest personal energy and time to gain depth of understanding of another person's life, as it is experienced, via life history.

THE PROBLEM

Incest has been described as a phenomenon that is morally abhorred, yet socially tolerated (Burgess, Groth, Holstrom, & Sgroi, 1978). It is much more common than society readily admits, with prevalence studies estimating 6% to 62% of women having been sexually abused during childhood (Finkelhor, 1987; Kinsey, Pomeroy, Martin, & Gebhard, 1953; Russell, 1983). In one of the more rigorous studies, Russell estimated that 20% of women experience at least one incestuous experience before age 18.

Estimating incidence and prevalence is problematic, in part owing to a wide variance in defining criteria utilized by investigators and a reluctance to report family crimes (Finkelhor, 1984; Wyatt & Peters, 1986). Legal use of the term most often considers sexual intercourse between closely related persons (forbidden to marry) as defining criteria (Black, 1979). Early studies used legal criteria for case identification (Kinsey et al., 1953; Landis, 1956).

States' statutes vary with regard to the actual relationship between participants and the degree of sexual activity required to meet the defining criteria for incest. All states recognize intercourse between blood relatives as being incestuous, but activities such as fondling and masturbation are not consistently addressed. Helping professionals have asserted that any form of sexual activity is incestuous when it occurs between family members, violates the trust of a caretaking relationship, and is inappropriate for the age of one or more of the participants (Forward & Buck, 1978; Justice & Justice, 1979; The National Center for the Prevention of Child Abuse and Neglect, 1981). Research literature reflects criteria for incest to include exhibitionism, pornography, fondling, masturbation, and oral-genital contact (Finkelhor, 1984; Russell, 1986; Wyatt & Peters, 1986) indulged in by extended family members such as adoptive or foster parents, stepparents, and significant others who occupy a caregiving role on which the victim is dependent (Grando, 1983; Gruber & Jones, 1983; Russell, 1984; Vander Mey & Neff, 1982, 1986).

Perceptions of sexual behavior within the family are culturally defined. Behavior considered incestuous in American culture is routinely practiced with positive sanctioning in other cultures. For example, males of an East African tribe routinely practice intercourse with their young daughters prior to a hunting expedition, believing the ritual will bring luck to the tribal hunt. Other cultures practice similar rituals (Goldman & Wheeler, 1986; Sgroi, 1988). The experience of incest within an approving environment is unknown. Sexual behavior that is positively sanctioned and free from cognitive dissonance may not be perceived as harmful (Henderson, 1983). Yet incest is believed to be universally taboo. Thus, if the tribesman engaged in cross-generational intercourse indiscriminately, the behavior would violate their cultural norms. The research literature has failed to assess the actual experience of the incest victim from the emic point of view. Janeway (1981) theorized the victim's experience as:

- The experience of exploitation by a powerful, older significant other to whom a child is affectionately indebted
- The incorporation of secrecy and shame into sexual interactions
- Distortion of a child's self-perception such that she views herself as a sexual object rather than as a multifaceted individual (p. 61).

Although victims may report having experienced no adverse effects (Constantine, 1980; Henderson, 1983; Koch, 1980), incest is believed to create lifelong sequelae for victims (Courtois, 1988; Crewdson, 1988; Haugaard & Reppucci, 1988; Jacobsen, 1986; Wyatt & Powell, 1988). An extensive review of theoretical and research literature has generated information about the injurious effects of incest (Browne & Finkelhor, 1986; Finkelhor, 1979, 1986, 1987; Friedrich, 1988; Friedrich, Urquiza, & Beilke, 1986; Goldman & Wheeler, 1986).

Repetition and reinforcement of incestuous dynamics and effects may occur when the victim is sexually exploited by a mental health professional (Burgess & Hartman, 1986). The incidence of sexual exploitation of female clients by male therapists has been estimated to range from 6.4% to 12.1% (Derosia, Hamilton, Morrison, & Strauss, 1987; Gartrell, Herman, & Olarte, 1986; Holroyd & Brodsky, 1977; Kluft, 1989; Pope & Bouhoutsos, 1986). Although appalling, these estimates are likely underestimated, as they are based on self-reports, and the actual number of offenses per therapist are unreported. Pope, Keith-Spiegel, and Tabachnik (1986) reported findings of a national survey of psychologists, which indicated that 87% reported experiencing sexual attraction to their clients, with 7% admitting acting on their attractions, and 18% considering doing so. The effect of sexualized therapy is believed to be detrimental to the patient's recovery (Burgess & Hartman, 1986; Kluft, 1989; Plasil, 1985; Pope & Bouhoustos, 1986; Walker, & Young, 1986).

Therapist–client sexual intimacy is recognized as a departure from acceptable practice, both by health care professionals and their Hippocratic origins (Pope & Bouhoutsos, 1986). Clients are extremely vulnerable to health care providers, as they allow therapists to enter their most private, emotional world, where vulnerabilities are rampant. Clients seek out therapists when they feel incapable of managing situations and are thus easily influenced by another's authoritative suggestions. For some, the ability to think, perceive, and remember clearly may be impaired, which further increases their vulnerability. Transference phenomena, which further empowers the therapist to influence the client, often occur in therapy. The very vulnerability that led to the formation of a therapeutic relationship may influence the client's ability to consent or refuse a therapist's sexual advances. Nurse–therapists are just beginning to realize the dynamics of incest and sexual exploitation by a mental health professional and the influence of such abuse on an individual's development and subsequent functioning (Burgess & Hartman, 1986; Cambell & Humphreys, 1984; Robinson, 1982).

Scant research is available regarding therapist–client sexual relationships, partly owing to the sensitive nature of the topic. Likewise, much of the incest research is quantitative and focuses on identification of cause-and-effect relationships. Most investigations have been designed from a reductionist, positivist paradigm, which is based on the following assumptions:

- Reality is singular and can be dissected and examined independent of the whole, with knowledge gained from a single component equaling knowledge of the whole.
- Investigators are capable of maintaining unquestionable objectivity in their execution of research.
- Findings of any single observation are both time and context free and thus generalizable.
- There are no effects without causes and no causes without effects.
- Research is value-free and unbiased.

Conversely, the naturalistic paradigm asserts that realities are multiple and constructed by humans in a holistic manner. Examining pieces of reality yields fractional insight, which cannot be considered representative of the whole. Humans construct their realities in a holistic fashion, and the whole differs from the mere sum of the parts. To gain genuine insight into multiple and divergent human realities, Lincoln and Guba (1985) advocate use of the naturalistic paradigm. Tenets of the naturalistic paradigm include:

- The knower and the known are inseparable in the naturalistic paradigm. The researcher–respondent relationship is one of interdependence. Respondents are influenced by researchers and researchers by respondents, both of which affect the object of study. All investigations contain a degree of subjectivity; in the naturalistic paradigm, these subjective views are openly noted for the readers' evaluation (Lincoln & Guba, 1985).
- Time may refute truth, as knowledge is both time and context bound. Naturalistic paradigm research seeks to obtain ideographic, tentative knowledge for certain times and contexts. Knowledge of phenomena cannot be assumed transferable to phenomena of a different context or time. Similarities may exist, but so will differences (Lincoln & Guba, 1985).
- Human behavior is complex, and seeking linear explanation is inadequate in gaining understanding of relationships. Entities are shaped through mutual interaction, and therefore, seeking cause-and-effect, linear relationships is futile. The goal of naturalistic paradigm research is to uncover plausible explanations, mutual influences, and circularity (Lincoln & Guba, 1985).

- All human inquiry is value laden. The selection of a problem for study, the governing paradigm for investigation, the context and method of investigation, and the interpretative meanings attributed to findings, represent areas of value influence. The researcher's values must be identified and addressed openly to provide a frame for readers to evaluate the research (Lincoln & Guba, 1985).

In summary, the naturalistic paradigm asserts human realities are constructed holistically, in multiple and varied constructs; subjectivity is inherent in investigations; and knowledge is limited by both time and context. Although it is the paradigm most congruent with the phenomena, naturalistic paradigm research in the area of incest is virtually nonexistent. The victim's perspective of the lived experience remains unknown. Therefore, this study used the naturalistic paradigm for inquiry into the lived experience of incest.

PURPOSE

The purpose of this study was to discover the subjective experience of incest and subsequent sexual exploitation by a therapist, through a historical examination of one survivor's life and the cultural context in which she lived through the experiences.

ASSUMPTIONS

The assumptions for this study were as follows:

- Implementation of the life history method will ascertain elements of another's subjective perception and interpretation of life experiences (Langness & Frank, 1981).
- The respondent is able to recollect, frame, and express the lived experience through a life history review (Field & Morse, 1985; Langness & Frank, 1981; Watson & Watson-Franke, 1985).
- Acknowledgment of the researcher's perspective regarding the phenomena of interest is essential for control of prejudgments in naturalistic investigations (Burns, 1989).
- The researcher is able to express, through the written word, the lived experience of the incest survivor.

RESEARCH QUESTION

The research question for this investigation was, What is the lived experience of the survivor of both incest and sexual exploitation by a therapist?

Definitions obtained from reviews of the research and theoretical literature include:

Incest: Any sexually oriented contact or exposure between members of a nuclear or extended family, which exploits a caretaking relationship by engaging a victim in sexual activities inappropriate for his or her present developmental level for the sexual arousal and/or gratification of one or more of the participants and endangers the physical and/or psychological well-being of the victim.

Survivor: An adult older than age 18, who endured incestuous abuse during childhood, according to his or her self-report.

Experience: Subjective encounters with others and the environment as they occur over the course of time and are expressed by the respondent.

Life history: A "retrospective account by the individual of his life in whole or part, in written or oral form, that has been elicited or prompted by another person" (Watson & Watson-Franke, 1985, p. 2).

SIGNIFICANCE

A qualitative assessment of the subjective experience of the incest survivor adds a new, thus-far omitted, dimension to nursing knowledge. As the actual experience of incest, as it is lived on a daily basis, is unknown, the discovery contributes to nursing's knowledge base and provides a foundation for theory development. Eliciting subjective meaning and reflection of lived experiences also reveals the values and beliefs of a particular cultural perspective (Ray, 1985). Findings of this study were analyzed to extract constructs, patterns, themes, and propositions, which will contribute to future theory building at the factor-isolating and factor-relating level.

Watson and Watson-Franke (1985) noted a dearth of women's life histories, and those in existence were implemented as supplements to male histories, evidencing an apparent cultural bias. Knowledge of cultural values and beliefs may influence health states, practices, and nursing's role in providing health care. Gaining insight into the meaning of an experience reveals the quality of existence and the health beliefs of an individual (Ray, 1985).

Lived experiences constitute concern for nursing within the context of client relation to health and to future functioning (Donaldson, 1987; Goochman, 1988; Leininger, 1985). An understanding and appreciation of the incest survivor's world is essential for the development of insightful, therapeutic interventions for victims and their families. The findings of this study generated information that can be used in the development of nursing interventions for survivors in the areas of primary, secondary, and tertiary prevention.

In the area of primary prevention, strategies to promote health, prevent illness, educate the community, and provision community resources are paramount. The goal is the prevention of illness through support. Strategies for anticipatory guidance, stress management, crisis intervention, and self-help are proposed from the findings of this study. Knowledge of measures that the subject views as helpful in aiding adaptation and coping is imperative to assist other potential victims through primary prevention measures. Identification of means of educating the public regarding ethical standards of practice and of training therapists to be sensitive to such issues in therapy are also addressed by this study.

Secondary prevention strategies, those aimed at reducing the prevalence of illness, are also generated by this study. Prompt and aggressive case finding, followed by rapid access to skilled treatment, are the goals of secondary prevention. Insight into the victim's experience, both of incest and of sexual exploitation by a mental health professional, are gained through this study. Assisting individuals to regain a sense of control by seeking legal recourse is also addressed and measures of positive influence identified. Treatment must be perceived as helpful by the client if it is to be effective, and the victim's perception of the nature and effect of treatment is illuminated by this study. Treatment often focuses on helping clients alter their environmental situations or learn new coping skills to deal with situations differently. Insight into the victim's perspective of the environment and ability to cope with situations yields strategies in the secondary prevention realm.

Tertiary prevention is oriented toward preventing complications and resocializing individuals to independence. Measures of ongoing support that may aid in adaptation are obtained through the holistic examination of the victim's experience. Therapeutic measures to assist incest victims and those sexually abused by mental health professionals are essential to prevent lifelong difficulties. Identifying strategies to assist clients to adapt and cope, without having abusive experiences consume their lives, is another expected benefit of this study.

METHODOLOGY

Design

The study design of this study was ethnographic, and therefore descriptive, as the purpose was to gain insight into the lived experience of an incest survivor. To provide a holistic examination of the subjective experience, the life history method was chosen. The life history method employs extensive interviewing and other techniques of inquiry to elicit the emic point of view, as the person is currently trying to make sense of his or her world (Watson & Watson-Franke, 1985). Detailed accounts of the development of an individual's life provide data for identifying common patterns experienced by the individual, which may also be experienced by their peers (Dobbert, 1982; Field & Morse, 1985).

Instrumentation

The primary means through which data were collected was unstructured interviews with the investigator serving as the instrument. Classical anthropology, as well as sociological field research, has rarely used any instrument other than the investigator (Lincoln & Guba, 1985). When conducting research in a naturalistic paradigm, it is virtually impossible to devise, a priori, an instrument that is sufficiently adaptable and comprehensive to address the encompassing realities that will be encountered (Lincoln & Guba, 1985).

As the investigator for this study, I was classically trained in the scientific method and reductionist paradigm. But as a clinician, I found research generated from a reductionist paradigm to be inadequate in examining the nuances of interpersonal phenomena in a holistic context. Interprofessional coursework and experiential learning in the naturalistic paradigm were sought and found to be more compatible with holistic human subject research. Guided experiential learning afforded me the opportunity to design and implement multiple, small-scale, qualitative investigations, practice measures to ensure data validity and reliability, gain skill in the interpretation of qualitative data, and practice eliciting the subjective viewpoint of lived experiences. As a nurse–therapist, I had clinical experience in the care of sexually abused clients and their families. I found data offered by research conducted in the reductionist paradigm to be inadequate in identifying difficulties experienced by survivors and in identifying therapeutic interventions to assist survivors adapt and cope. Having experience with incest survivors, I noted a divergent range of functioning, experiences, and perceptions expressed by survivors, a phenomenon not yet represented in research or theoretical literature.

As the investigator, I was the primary instrument in this ethnographic study. Other tools included an unstructured interview guide to focus the questions, a life story critical incident chart, and a description of the respondent's family.

Rigor

Traditional reductionist measures of reliability and validity of instrumentation are not applicable to naturalistic paradigm research. There are, however, correlates to address rigor of the human instrument. Validity of data depends on prolonged engagement or time of sufficient duration and intensity to gain understanding (Lincoln & Guba, 1985). An investigator's lack of self-awareness can also drastically alter data collection and analysis. As human instruments, investigators bring with them biases from their own culture, experiences, personalities, and theoretical commitments that must be not only acknowledged but also consciously examined to evaluate their influence on data collection and interpretation.

As the gathering of data for a life history involves ongoing interchange between the investigators and the respondents, the personality of the investigator may influence the respondent's disclosure. Prior to data collection and throughout the process, I examined my cultural and theoretical bias, personal beliefs and values, personality characteristics, and communication techniques. The context of data collection was social, open, and emotionally charged. I was often angered by the respondent's life experiences and awed by her inner strength and wisdom. Following data collection and during data analysis, these issues were readdressed and efforts made to separate emic from etic views. Data, recorded and interpreted, were reviewed by the respondent during the analysis phase to ensure approximation to the respondent's view of the world. Editing of the final product was minimal but identifying characteristics were altered to protect the identity of the respondent.

Sample: Amy

The purposive sample consisted of one adult female (Amy is a pseudonym) who had a history of incestuous abuse and subsequent exploitation by a therapist. A female was selected because the research literature reflects that females are more commonly victims of incest and therapist sexual abuse (Burgess & Hartman, 1986; Finkelhor, 1984; Herman & Hirschman, 1981). There are several ethical considerations inherent to this method of sampling. The person had to be willing to voluntarily disclose, examine, and reconstruct the meanings of her life; she was informed of the design, procedure, time commitment, and potential risks and benefits of participation. Strategies to equalize the power between the respondent and the investigator included the use of informed consent, respondent review of the data, and exclusion of my current and prior clients of the nurse–therapist from eligibility, as described by Chenitz and Swanson (1986). A pseudonym was assigned to protect the respondent from identification.

Procedures

Prior to data collection, permission was obtained from the institutional review board of the university where I had registered as a doctoral student. Unstructured interviews were conducted and audiotaped. Audiotaping enabled me to provide undivided attention and closely observe and process the respondent without the interruption or distraction of note-taking. Although it was impossible to realize, a priori, the specific questions, a sampling of potential questions was compiled and served as tools to focus if the respondent did not voluntarily address a topic. Sufficient time was spent eliciting demographic and other general information prior to inquiring about abusive incidents and relationships to facilitate trust and subject comfort.

Unstructured interview focused on gaining insight into the respondent's view of what was relevant to be shared. Questioning was paced to move from general to specific and from impersonal to personal. The length of each interview varied and was controlled by the respondent. Interview sessions were held in my home and respondents' homes, at the respondent's convenience. Prior to terminating each interview, I summarized the interview. The respondent was invited to react to the summary of the interview session by remarking on the validity of my constructions, thereby providing a member check for validity of the information obtained. Summation also induced the respondent to elaborate on certain points (Lincoln & Guba, 1985). Following each interview, audiotapes were transcribed into notes. Transcription was performed by me to prevent potential voice identification of the respondent. Audiotapes, field notes, and the consent form were maintained in a locked cabinet in my home. Following completion of the study, audiotapes were destroyed by the researcher. Verbatim transcription occurred as soon as feasible, and notations regarding the emotional atmosphere, nonverbal cues, and environmental factors perceived by me were added and correlated with the verbatim content.

Efforts to assess reliability and validity were exerted during the data collection phase including prolonged engagement, persistent observation, member checks, and triangulation. The informant was asked for the same information at repeated intervals, as advocated by Langness and Frank (1981). This allowed me to assess the reliability of the information provided. A typical technique utilized to attain these data is to inquire about a topic discussed previously as if asking for clarification, such as, "I know we have discussed this before, but I am not certain that I understand, could you tell me about it again?" Information provided was then compared with that previously elicited to assess reliability.

Measures to enhance credibility and internal validity of data included use of prolonged engagement, persistent observation, member checks, and triangulation. Prolonged engagement is an investment of time to achieve an appreciation of the culture, testing for misinformation, and building trust. More than 30 hours were spent with the respondent, and respondent reviews were used to establish credibility.

Triangulation involves the use of multiple sources of the same information. Supplemental data, such as court records, depositions, and newspaper clippings, were used to acquire as much information as possible about the individual and the environment in which the experiences occurred. Supplemental data also offered validation of the subjective information provided. The respondent was given an opportunity to correct or clarify information and assess the overall adequacy of the data in representing her construction of reality.

Persistent observation involves identification of those elements that are most relevant to the focus of the investigation and focusing on these to gain depth of understanding. Pervasive qualities of the respondent's experience were identified and separated from less pertinent points. The investigator engaged in tentative labeling of salient factors and explored those in depth in subsequent interviews. Field notes were used to chart salient features and record how salient features were identified and isolated to form an auditable trail of data collection decisions.

Member checks were used by having the respondent review the data recorded for validity and approximation to her subjective experience. An opportunity to correct or clarify information and assess the overall adequacy of the data in representing her construction of reality was given. Member checks provided throughout the data collection process also provided the respondent with an opportunity to further process her experience.

The data collection phase concluded when historical and conceptual saturation occurred, in other words, when the information offered by the respondent became redundant. Data collection ceased after the respondent replied, "I can't think of anything else to tell you." Termination of the investigator and respondent relationship in life history research, in which sharing of personal details and feelings occurs over a period of time, can be difficult (Chenitz & Swanson, 1986). Strategies typically employed for the termination of a therapeutic relationship were utilized to aid closure for both the respondent and the investigator.

Each step of the investigation was documented, creating an audit trail, or a methodological log of the process of inquiry was produced and included the following: (a) raw data such as field notes and transcriptions; (b) data reduction products such as coding categories; (c) data synthesis products, such as themes, interpretations, and inferences made by the researcher; (d) process notes such as procedures, strategies, and rationales for choices and decisions made; and (e) intention notes such as personal reflective notes and preliminary interpretations.

Data Analysis

A series of analysis strategies were implemented to systematically extrapolate meaning from the data. Techniques began concretely, progressed to the conceptual, and included unitizing, noting patterns, categorizing, noting relations, and building conceptual coherence (Lincoln & Guba, 1985; Miles & Huberman, 1984). Data were first separated into individual units. Units consisted of the smallest possible piece of information about something that can have meaning in the absence of additional information. More than 1,000 data units were entered onto index cards and each card coded according to the interview during which the unit was collected and the source of the data (respondent, court record, newspaper clipping, etc.).

After isolating units of data, the next step was pattern noting. Through repeated data review, frequently repeated themes, explanations, constructs, or relationships emerged. Themes that emerged were identified and word labels chosen that represent the category of information. Categories are collections of cards that relate to the same content or property. Rules were devised to justify inclusion of cards (data units) into a category and to provide internal consistency for the set. The initial step in categorization was to select the first card from the complete set of unitized cards. The first card was read, noting its content, and set aside. The next card was read and its contents evaluated as to whether it is alike, in content or emotion, to the first card. If it was similar, it was added to the first card stack; if dissimilar, a new, separate category was begun. Each successive card was assessed, comparing and contrasting the data unit with prior categories. Each card that contained a unit of data that differed from the prior categories was set aside to begin a new category (Lincoln & Guba, 1985; Miles & Huberman, 1984).

The goal of the noting relations phase of data analysis was creating homogeneous categories. I read and reread data units to discern dissimilarities within the categories and explore other plausible themes. Repeated reviews of the categories aided in recognition of data that "just do not fit" the scheme, which were then removed, and either entered into a different category, or became a new category. This process continued until all of the data fit homogeneously into categories (Lincoln & Guba, 1985; Miles & Huberman, 1984).

To build conceptual coherence, categories were reexamined with the following question in mind, What commonalities do the units of a category share? Commonalities, once identified, were at a more abstract level than the preliminary category labels. At this point, a construct label that depicts the content and emotion of the category was selected. The construct label was one that captured the theme or essence of the category. The constructs identified contribute to factor-isolation, for the construction of factor-isolating and factor-relating theory in subsequent studies. As a final means of exerting trustworthiness and rigor, the construct-labels were reviewed by the respondent to ascertain representativeness or validity with her lived experience.

Limitations

1. As the investigator, I was a novice in implementing the life history, and this may have influenced the process and product.
2. I reviewed the literature on incest and therapist sexual exploitation a priori, and, therefore, may have been biased by other etic viewpoints.
3. Audiotaping may have inhibited disclosure.
4. A hermeneutical gap between the emic and etic perspectives and meanings may have existed.

RESULTS

The results of this study are summarized. Because the original version of this chapter was a dissertation, the results were too detailed to include in the scope of this work. As data were collected, analysis proceeded and raw data were categorized into a typology of concepts and themes. The original dissertation included 23 themes with a number of direct quotes from Amy that illustrated the themes in the life story of a woman incestuously abused and sexually exploited by a therapist. Several themes that illustrate the strengths and positive outcomes experienced by the respondent, themes virtually absent in the incest literature of the time, emerged. The themes identified were as follows: anger, control, loss, betrayal, guilt, magical thinking, powerlessness, rescuing others, need to belong, retreat, fantasy, unreasonable expectations, cultural sanctions, diffuse boundaries, risk taking, ambivalence, affirmation of value, tenacity, assertion, insight, acceptance, appreciation, and hope. These themes were often concurrent, sequential, and/or interrelated. Several of these themes are summarized in the following sections.

Amy's Story

Amy is a petite woman of 5 feet 2 inches with an energetic smile and demeanor. Her appearance is neat, and her dress is fashionable. She resides in a small rural town where neighbors know each other. Her home is decorated with the details that make a house feel like a home: photos of her children, crafts, and toys. Her parents attended grade school together and married immediately after high school. In the rural farm community where they grew up, it was expected, as a cultural norm, that young high school graduates marry and begin a family. Instead of going to college, people went to work in factories or family farms.

> For my mother's generation at this time, in this town, to try to presume to even go to college was just pretentious.

Born 9 months after her parents' marriage, Amy is the oldest of four children. Thirteen months later, her younger brother was born. Her parents' inexperience and youth contributed to what Amy remembers as difficult parenting.

> I think a whole lot of what happened when I was young was related to the fact that they were very young and my father was just not ready. It's not like they had time to adjust to one baby before they had another, and he just couldn't handle it.

Ten and 12 years later, two more children were born in the family. Amy recalled her parents' skills as being markedly different with her young siblings.

My father says had he become a father again now, he'd be damn good at it.

Until recently, Amy blamed herself for the difficulties the family experienced when she was a child.

I had been focusing on "What did I do wrong?" and "What was wrong with me that you couldn't do it right?" and I finally realized they did the best that they could.

Her mother is introverted, preferring solitary activities such as reading romance novels. She described her father as an intelligent man who never had the opportunity to attend college and thus has spent his life farming and working in factories. With vivid detail, Amy recalled a traumatic experience she had at the age of 3. She was hospitalized for a tonsillectomy and recalled the nightgown she wore, playing with the nurses, and then being taken from her mother's arms to the operating room. The rebellion of a frightened child is evident in her recollection.

The nurse reached for me and I was screaming. This was something I did not want to do and "leave me alone, I am not going," and I was physically pried off my mother. I remember the ether mask being put over my face and the nurse saying "doesn't it smell like roses? Just smell the pretty roses" and I thought, "I hate roses, I hate roses. This doesn't smell like roses!"

Most of her preschool days were spent playing with her brother on the family farm. She remembers her mother would allow the two children to play in the fields even though they would always end up splashing about in the mud. There is a history of abuse in the extended family. Amy's maternal great-grandfather and great uncles were notoriously abusive. Through the generations, daughters and granddaughters were warned to avoid these men.

It was just understood, you don't hug grandpa and you darn sure don't hug him alone. All of the female cousins, they're all mental wrecks today. It was just real common.

She remembered her great-grandmother hiding her from him.

She bodily stood in front of me while I hovered in a corner because grandpa was after me. I can't remember what for, but he was angry, and he wanted me out of there. And I was a very small child.

When he died, her great-grandmother, and the entire family, felt a sense of relief.

The family's farmhand had a son about the same age as Amy's brother. The three played together out of necessity; there were no other children for miles. One day while playing, the farmhand grabbed Amy and took her into the bedroom and locked the door. She recalled being both frightened and confused. He removed her panties, touched her genitalia, and exposed himself to her.

I remember thinking, "that doesn't look anything like my brother!" It was terrible.

He tried to force her to perform fellatio, and she bit him. He shoved her away and left angrily. She recalled feeling angry that her brother had continued playing outside, yet she never told him what happened. Thereafter she avoided the farmhand. She did not disclose this abuse to anyone for more than 20 years.

She began school the next year and developed friendships. When she was 7, her maternal grandparents divorced and her grandmother left the home and her two children with Amy's grandfather. The two children, a boy and a girl were technically her uncle and aunt, but were only 5 years older than Amy. She recalled her grandfather was ill prepared to care for the two children. One evening he had been drinking and fondled his 12-year-old daughter. The daughter, Sue, protested and complained to her older sister, Amy's mother. Soon after, both of the children came to live with Amy's family. Although one of the children, Sam, would return to live with his father within a year, the other child, her aunt Sue, remained with Amy's family. Sue suddenly became the oldest child of the family, a position Amy felt belonged to her. The sibling rivalry between the two became fierce. Amy remembered her mother spoiling Sue, which her mother openly admitted. Amy also recalled being jealous of Sue's assertiveness; telling her father to stop touching her and complaining to her older sister, who then rescued her.

I was so jealous, because she had said, "don't do that" and it was fixed. She didn't care if it was okay, whose fault it was, or anything. She knew it was wrong and she stopped it. I just felt so jealous.

The family moved when Amy was in the middle of the third grade. She hated leaving her friends and the people she had known her entire life. Her father was having a difficult time supporting the family by farming and moved them to a nearby city where he had found work in a factory. Owing to changes being made in the school district, Amy changed schools three times that year. With the frequent changes, she had difficulty establishing friendships. Although her mother and 5-years-older aunt were in the home, she recalls both being more self-absorbed than interested in Amy. She remembered caring for herself and her younger brother.

> No one picked out clothes for me to wear to school, I just dressed myself. I remember a cafeteria worker making fun of me and saying, "Doesn't this child have a mother?" cause I had worn a sleeveless jumper to school in the dead of winter.

The attention she missed at home was sought in the classroom.

> I would bond with every school teacher I had. I was up in their face: "here I am, notice me." I guess they knew I did that cause I wasn't recognized at home.

She remembered being domineering and bossy with the other children, who often came to her for instructions. A cousin of Amy's, who was also a childhood playmate, told her how domineering and intimidating she really was. Amy and her cousin were born 3 months apart, so the two were frequently compared to each other at family gatherings. Amy was regarded as the pretty one and her cousin as withdrawn, quiet, and awkward. Yet Amy idealized her cousin, who possessed artistic talents and wealth. Amy stated she found it ironic that she would envy her cousin so much, as family comments often focused on Amy's beauty and popularity, when she really wanted to be like her cousin. As adults her cousin told her of an incident in which Amy used a pair of scissors to threaten her cousin, forcing her to play with her. Amy did not remember the incident but did recall intimidating children on the playground and wanting to control others.

While in the fifth grade, Amy accidentally discovered that the farmhand who had abused her also lived nearby. His son rode the same school bus Amy and her brother rode. This frightened her because she had not recognized his son and she thought he might have followed her. She fantasized of killing him with fuel her father kept in storage.

> I remember thinking it would be fun to kill him. I remember thinking about the fuel my father kept with the equipment and that I could sneak into his house and set his house on fire and nobody would know it was me. Nobody would ever know, but I wanted him to know who killed him.

She was abused again while in the sixth grade. Her Uncle Sam and her grandfather lived nearby. Her uncle, 5 years her senior, had a motorcycle that she enjoyed riding. Sam would lure her to the barn under the pretense of riding the motorcycle, then kiss and fondle her. He threatened to tell her mother as coercion and continued to abuse her periodically for about a year. When Amy's mother became pregnant, Amy asked if she too would become pregnant if touched in her genital region. Suspicious, her mother confronted Sam who ceased abusing Amy.

She remembered the sixth grade as a critical point in her life, a time of decisions and choices. She had to choose between continuing athletics or pursuing new skills in dance and piano. She felt confident that athletics were the right choice for her until she entered junior high.

> I should've taken piano and dance and all those other things because I wasn't going to make it in sports.

Amy's friends nominated her to compete in a beauty pageant. She recalled feeling inferior to the other contestants because she did not possess a talent acceptable for the pageant competition.

> All my girlfriends that had gone to ballet and dance and stuff and were just the perfect ladies, they were so ladylike and feminine. I can remember being voted to be in the young beauty pageant and having no talent, because you don't mount a tetherball and call someone up from the audience to impress them, you just don't.

She did compete but remembered the experience as humiliating and degrading and refused to participate in future pageants.

Amy's younger siblings, 10 and 12 years younger, were born and her father sought work in a larger city. The family moved again in time for Amy to begin the seventh grade in another new school. She longed for her old friends and the school where she felt important. They moved into a poorer neighborhood near the railroad tracks. When school began in the fall, Amy had to ride city transit buses to junior high school while her brother walked to an elementary school nearby. Riding the city buses was traumatic. The passengers fondled the young girls when they boarded and left the bus. Fighting was frequent on the bus, and Amy prayed fervently,

> Dear God, I don't care what it takes, get me back home.

As the aggression on the bus intensified, Amy became more fearful, passive, and withdrawn. One day, on the trip home, Amy's cousin Cheryl was sitting with her boyfriend, arguing with another girl on the bus. Suddenly, the girl put a knife to the boyfriend's throat. She held the boyfriend at bay while several men raped Cheryl. The rape took place in the back of the bus, in front of onlookers, most of whom were participating, cheering the attack, or both.

> I didn't know what rape was until I saw it and I knew. It's just one of those things you know when you're seeing it.

Amy began screaming, which led the bus driver to stop and inquire as to what was the problem. One of the men told Amy, "you're next blondie, say it and you're next." Amy sat silent, confident he meant what he had said. Cheryl fled the bus at the next stop. When Amy's stop approached, she was afraid to move, but she was thrown from the bus by one of the men. She noticed that Cheryl's boyfriend had not been allowed to leave the bus. She remembered thinking: "They're going to kill him; they're going to cut his throat and he's going to die." Once home, the shock of what she had witnessed began to diminish. She wanted to tell someone, but felt she could not. She remembered crying, being angry, and yelling. She realized she was not behaving as usual, but did not understand why.

> I didn't eat, and I can remember just sitting there looking at everybody like, "why don't you know that something's not right" and "why don't you know what's happened today?" I was mad. I woke up screaming through the night. And I remember my mother saying, "I don't know what's going on with you, but you've got to get over this."

The next morning, she faked illness and stayed home from school.

> I'd never stayed home from school by myself and here I was in this Black neighborhood. But I knew that anything that could happen to me in that house alone was better than getting on that bus again.

She smoked her first cigarette on this day, hoping it would make her feel better. It did not. That evening, at the dinner table, she blurted, "Cheryl was raped on the bus." Amy recalled her father promptly left the room, while her mother questioned her. This was the first Amy had told her mother of the violence and abuse she had experienced on the bus. Her mother notified the police, who came to their home to question Amy. Like her mother, the police officer asked Amy, "Do you know what rape is?" Before she could respond, her mother interrupted, "I know she knows what it means, but whether it happened or not. . . ." Amy felt betrayed that her own mother doubted her. The officer furthered his investigation by questioning Cheryl. He later returned to talk with Amy and told her that there had been no rape and that there may have been roughhousing, but Cheryl denied being raped. He told her that "sometimes you see things that aren't really so." Amy was angered that no one believed her, and instead, they had rationalized her behavior as a response to the bus violence.

> I remember my mother telling him that one of the boys had "touched my private bottom" or "rubbed up against my chest" and she thought that was what was so upsetting to me. So they just decided between them that I had like made this up because some kid had touched my butt.

Her parents decided to move Amy and her brother back to the country, where the two lived with their paternal grandparents. Her grandfather was an alcoholic, and the two children learned that when he was drinking he would give them money to get rid of them. She adapted readily to the new environment but retained a sense of betrayal that no one had believed her report of the sexual assault of her cousin. While living in the city, she had longed for her old friends. She had expected her friends would welcome her with open arms, but she found her friends had carried on without her.

> I was glad to be where I was but it wasn't the same. I remember think-ing "ya'll aren't making this easy. Ya'll should just fall all over me now that I'm back and make me feel like what I used to be."

She felt like an outsider in what had been her hometown.

> I wasn't supposed to be an outsider there. I could understand being an outsider in the city but not in my home school.

A social studies teacher befriended Amy. He offered her his time and atten-tion when her old friends ignored her. She recalled the relationship as friendly and supportive.

> He treated me like a friend, not like a kid.

She spent time talking with him before and after school. She remem-bered thinking he knew what had happened to her in the city, although she did not recall telling him. The relationship was short-lived. Several of the other girls were envious of Amy's relationship with the teacher and began spreading rumors. The girls teased and taunted her until the tension between them rose to a climax. The girls were caught passing a note about Amy and the social studies teacher. The note insinuated the two were engaged in a sexual relationship. All of the girls, including Amy, were sent to the guidance office for counseling. The school board investigated, and the teacher resigned at the end of the school year. Amy did not learn of the circumstances of his resignation until years later.

That summer, the family moved again and Amy was given the responsibility of babysitting her younger siblings, who were 1 and 3 years old. When she handled this responsibility, she was given more household duties until she was soon fulfilling the homemaker role. She recalls her younger siblings came to her for permission, help, and nurturing. She recalled during this summer, she had her career aspirations crushed. Amy had hoped to attend college and pursue a career in either journalism or architecture. A relative inquired, at a family gathering, about her plans after high school. Amy began describing what she planned to study in college. Her mother interrupted to say, "Well, I don't think that you've really got a choice since you're not going to be going." Her mother proceeded to inform Amy that the family could not afford college, and therefore she could just forget about going.

In the fall, Amy began the eighth grade in a new school and was received very well by her peers. She met another new girl, who became a close friend. One of the most popular kids in school gave a party early in the school year. Everyone was invited except the new kids, Amy and her friend, Lisa. Lisa convinced Amy to crash the party. Although anxious, Amy agreed and was awed by her new friend's social skill. After crashing the party, the two became popular, an attribute important to Amy.

> I guess that struck chord with these other kids, that we had the chutzpa to do that because I can remember school the next week and we were it, we had made it. And I still believe that crashing that party was what made the difference. We could have been the girls that were on the outside, or we could run with the main crew, and this is what did it for us.

Amy's first sustained relationship with a boy began in the ninth grade. The two dated for several years and she remembered him as "a good kid, someone I trusted." As the intimacy and trust of their relationship grew, she recalled considering venturing into a sexual relationship with him but never disclosed if she acted on her desires.

Although she recalled junior high was a happy time, high school was different. Amy was not accepted by her peers, and she felt isolated and depressed much of the time. She recalled a marked change in her dress, mood, and friends. She spent more time alone, in solitary activities such as embroidery. She often retreated to her room and listened to melancholic music. She shared a bedroom with her older aunt and recalled she would sit in a closet for privacy.

> Sometimes the bedroom just wasn't isolated enough, and I would get in the far corner of my closet and stay there and do nothing. I can remember my mother finding me sitting in the closet one time, and it really distressed her, and I just thought, "what's it to you?"

After her mother found her in the closet, she began retreating to the attic.

A friend introduced Amy to marijuana. She remembered fearing her life was destined for skid row when she first began smoking marijuana. The fear did not materialize, but Amy's social circles did change. She found herself on the outside, no longer a member of the popular group. She was no longer elected for homecoming, and her friends changed. Although popularity had been important to her in the past, she no longer felt it was worth the effort. She chose to hang out with the smokers but soon felt uncomfortable with them as well. Amy found herself isolated and felt she could not return to her old friends. Amy's mood was labile during this time. She remembered being sensitive to other's cues and responding to them emotionally.

> Somebody could look at me crooked, and I would just spend the whole day crying: I was just so depressed!

At 16, Amy lost her virginity to a boyfriend she thought loved her. They met in the spring and dated throughout the summer. He attended a different high school, so, as the summer drew to a close, they realized they would not be seeing each other as often.

> So, in the fall, we decided this is the time, this is what we want to do. And I didn't see him again. Again I was just used. And it was just so like everything I'd ever known. He was on the basketball team and decided he needed a girlfriend that was a cheerleader. And that just about killed me. It took me a long time to get over it, and I don't think I am over that still.

Soon afterward, she attempted suicide. Her parents found her and took her to the emergency room. After gavage and stabilization, a sheriff's deputy questioned her. When she refused to talk to him, he informed her that she had broken the law. She found his attitude ironic, as jail was not where she had planned to go. The discomfort of the suicide attempt surprised her.

Amy encountered an old acquaintance, Bill, at a local ball game and he asked her to dinner. Amy and Bill had attended high school together. He was a year older, and the two had shared mutual friends in high school but never dated. Amy described Bill as "a hippy, pseudo educated type" when they began dating. Their dating relationship continued until Bill moved to a nearby town owing to job relocation. After graduating high school, Amy decided to move in with Bill, and they soon married.

Amy took a part-time retail job but felt the customers of the clothing store insulted her by treating her as a child. She quit the job and returned to homemaking. She began what she referred to as "nesting" by baking bread, sewing, and talking about babies, which she recalled made Bill very nervous. He encouraged her to enroll in a practical nurse program, which she did.

As a young couple, one of their first social contacts led them to reconsider socializing. They developed a friendship with a couple who were 10 years older than Bill and Amy. The couple was socially prominent in their small town, and Bill and Amy were flattered to be included in their social circles. They were invited to a dinner party at another couple's home. Once there, it became clear the couples were interested in mate swapping. Bill and Amy excused themselves and returned home, a little less venturesome into the small town's social events.

Amy's menstrual periods became increasingly painful and Amy avoided intercourse, complaining of pain. Bill told her the problem was psychological, and Amy thought he might be right. She realized she had never really enjoyed sex.

> That was probably the first time that I became conscious that I had a problem with sex and with intimacy, with everything. But the pain was real to me.

She scheduled an appointment with a reputable gynecologist in a nearby city. The pelvic exam was intensely painful and the physician insensitive. He bluntly told her that she had severe endometriosis, she would never have children, and that he recommended a hysterectomy. Amy was only 20 years old, and because she was in nursing school, he agreed to postpone the hysterectomy until she graduated. He prescribed birth control pills, which he advised her to take continuously to suppress menstruation. He advised Amy to return for surgery as soon as she finished school or sooner if the pain became intolerable. She was devastated, as she had always pictured herself as a mother.

Amy expected Bill to be relieved when he learned they would not be having children. Instead Bill threw the birth control pills away and had Amy consult her nursing instructor about monitoring her temperature to detect ovulation. They searched the literature for tips on conception, charted Amy's temperature, and tried everything they heard of or read about. She never returned to the gynecologist who gave her the birth control pills. She recalls each month when her period began, she felt like dying. After 5 months of trying, Amy noticed her breasts were swollen and painful. She was convinced she had willed the changes in her body. A urine specimen revealed her pregnancy. She was near graduation in the practical nurse program and was felt pressured by the faculty to quit, but she refused and successfully completed the program.

After she became pregnant, Bill was promoted to the position of regional manager and was required to travel away from home more. After graduation, Amy worked as a licensed practical nurse in a nursing home. She found the work routine and boring, giving medications and charting the same comments night after night. As her pregnancy progressed, she quit work. Near the end of her eighth month of pregnancy, the baby dropped, and she dilated 4 centimeters. Amy was ready. Her water broke 2 weeks before her due date. She woke Bill, who informed her he was going to work and to call him if her contractions started. By mid-morning her contractions had begun; she would give birth 3 hours later. Amy felt prepared for labor but was surprised by the intensity of her pain. Amy's obstetrician was not available, so another physician helped Amy relax by using visualization and hypnotizing her. Thereafter, she tolerated the labor pains, her labor progressed rapidly, and she delivered a healthy baby. Throughout her pregnancy, Amy had been certain the baby was a girl. When her son was born, she was obviously disappointed.

I needed a girl, a girl child that I could be comfortable with, that I wouldn't be afraid of. Recognizing her disappointment, the obstetrician helped her position herself for breastfeeding, assisted her in holding the child, and assessed her bonding with the infant over the course of several hours. She credited this physician with helping her bond with her new baby and recognize the importance of helping new mothers.

Amy did not return to work but stayed home with baby Mark. She recalled enjoying being home with Mark and fulfilling the role she has always envisioned for herself. On baby Mark's first birthday, Amy and Bill decided to try to conceive again. Again they used temperature charts and a year later became successful. On her first prenatal visit, she was again told the severity of her endometriosis warranted a hysterectomy. Eight months into this pregnancy Amy felt something was wrong. The office staff tried to convince her she was overreacting, but at her insistence, they agreed to examine her. They found she had dilated to 5 centimeters. The next morning Amy went into labor. At noon the labor room nurse examined Amy and found she had dilated to 6 centimeters. Half an hour later Amy called the nurse complaining of a need to push, but the nurse ignored her complaint.

She was obnoxious, she said, "we just checked you, you don't need to push, you need to relax."

Amy turned to Bill and told him the baby was coming; he believed her and changed into scrub clothes. Amy suddenly felt nauseated, vomited, and the baby was born precipitously. Chaos ensued.

The nurse was yelling and screaming at me because I had pushed without her telling me I could and who did I think I was and didn't I know that was dangerous. Bill had to lift me because I was scared to death of crushing the baby and I still hadn't delivered the placenta and I was all twisted. And the doctor wasn't there and the baby was just lying there turning blue. I thought I had killed my baby. I did not push, I vomited.

She recalled her room was suddenly filled with nurses, nursing students, medical residents, and even a visiting preacher. She had tears from the precipitous birth and was in pain. She remembers the entire experience as being terribly traumatic. After Amy and her new son, David, were discharged from the hospital, she continued to experience cramping. A week later she expelled a retained piece of placenta and subsequently experienced heavy bleeding. Although she reported this to the physician, he did not believe her. She tried to convince him to repair the tearing that had occurred during birth, but he claimed he saw nothing out of the ordinary. She recalled being forced to tolerate pain and chafing for years before she found a physician who finally recognized and repaired the tear.

Amy soon became increasingly aware of her anger toward men. She grew fearful of her children and herself.

I was scared to death of them. I had no business with children; it was a freak of nature that I had children and that I had "male" children was even more absurd. How dare God entrust me with male children. I was going to make rapists out of them. What else could I raise?

Her affect and behavior affected her parenting skills. Mark began having behavioral problems at preschool. Bill knew nothing of the abuse Amy experienced as a child and did not understand her mood swings. Both Amy and Bill recognized the family needed help, and the family, as a whole, sought professional guidance. Amy had met a counselor, who was also a minister, while she had been working part-time at the hospital. He often treated patients who were hospitalized on the floor where Amy had worked. The counselor, Mike, was still working under supervision. Mike's undergraduate study had been in religion and drama and his master's work in counseling. He was an ordained minister and a deacon in a local church. Although he had not completed the degree requirements for a doctorate in counseling education, he was licensed as a psychological examiner.

Amy made an appointment for the family with Mike. Following a 45-minute interview with the family, Mike identified the difficulty as stemming from Amy and explained Mark's behavior was merely in imitation of Amy's. They agreed that Amy would begin weekly therapy sessions. The goal of Amy's initial sessions with Mike was anger control. Although controlling her anger seemed to be the problem, actually it was merely a symptom of underlying conflicts. Amy wanted a simple answer, and regaining control of her life through controlling her anger, seemed to be the goal. Mike was supportive and told Amy what she yearned to hear, that she had value and worth. He identified her most pressing need, the need for approval and acceptance. Once he began meeting her needs, she became dependent on him.

At this time, Amy also learned that the family would be moving to another state in 3 months, as Bill had accepted a new job. Mike reported his assessment, goals, and treatment strategies for Amy in his weekly supervision sessions. Because Amy was to be moving soon, Mike's supervisor cautioned him not to delve too deeply in Amy's issues, as there was too little time to resolve any conflicts. Mike suggested administering the Minnesota Multiphasic Personality Inventory (MMPI) to Amy, but the supervisor discouraged him and again advised Mike to limit his sessions and goals with Amy and refer her to a therapist in the state where her family would soon be relocating.

Instead of following his supervisor's advice, Mike administered the MMPI to Amy and increased the frequency of their appointments to twice weekly. Amy trusted him and little by little began telling him of the abuses she experienced as a child. The more she disclosed to Mike, the more positive feedback and reinforcement he gave her. Amy felt relieved to finally ventilate the secrets she had kept hidden for so long.

> It just felt like such a relief, such immediate gratification to get so much off my chest, that I had kept hidden for so many years, and not be judged.

She recalled she had always felt dirty and evil and assumed others would blame her for her abuses. The relief she felt when Mike failed to blame her but instead reinforced how strong and wonderful he thought she was served to strengthen her bond to him.

At Mike's next supervision session, he mentioned Amy's MMPI results. Again his supervisor recommended he refer Amy, not only owing to her impending move, but also owing to transference issues. The supervisor believed Amy had begun to perceive Mike as the all-good, all-forgiving father figure. Instead of following his supervisor's advice, Mike continued to treat Amy biweekly and simply never mentioned her to the supervisor again. Mike also began hugging Amy, which he called physical comfort. When Amy saw how well Mike responded to her disclosures, she wanted to tell Bill also. She recalled Mike discouraged her from doing this and eventually convinced her not to tell Bill.

He didn't want me to tell anybody the stuff I had told him; he just didn't think that would be appropriate. And a part of me at that point said, "why wouldn't I want to do that? This is who I'm married to, the one who has to live with my mood swings from day to day. This is who's paying, this is who I would most like to have give me what you've given me, which is the sense of still having value that I never thought I had."

Amy pushed Mike to tell her the results of the MMPI he had administered. He resisted, but she persisted. Finally, he told her she was a little paranoid. Although still curious, she also feared the results indicated she was more seriously ill than she had thought. She would not fully discover the results for another year and a half.

She recalled in early May, Mike initiated sexual contact with her. He had gradually increased physical contact with her over the course of 2 months. Mike portrayed himself as a sexual surrogate, teaching Amy about male anatomy and desensitizing her to sexual contact. The evening following his initial sexual contact, Amy attempted suicide by overdosing with Xanax. A general practitioner had prescribed Xanax for Amy, at Mike's recommendation, as he thought Amy needed medication to control her anxiety.

Bill was out of town at the time but found Amy incoherent when he telephoned. She told him she had taken a bottle of Xanax. Frightened, Bill telephoned her therapist for advice. Mike convinced Bill that Amy would survive and that her suicidal gesture was evidence of the need for continued therapy sessions to resolve her childhood issues.

He told Bill, "you're going to have to make her come. If you care about her you have to make her come to therapy."

Amy pleaded with Bill that she did not want to return but was too fearful to tell him about Mike's sexual behavior. But Mike had already warned Bill that Amy might lie or make excuses to avoid returning to therapy. Amy had previously praised Mike for the help he had given her. Bill therefore believed that Mike had helped Amy and valued his professional opinion. Out of a desire to do what he could to help his wife, Bill forced Amy to return to the therapy appointments with Mike. Amy recalls thinking Bill's insistence was evidence of an agreement between her husband and Mike and that she was to cooperate with Mike's form of therapy. She returned to Mike's office.

She recalled Mike's sexual behavior escalated from kissing and fondling to exhibitionism, having Amy perform masturbation and fellatio and eventually, intercourse. He instructed her not to wear underwear to his office and had her meet him outside of the office. He maintained that his behavior was therapeutic with the goal being sexual desensitization.

As planned, in mid-June, the family moved to another state. Amy terminated the sessions with Mike, but he contacted her several times and requested she continue to see him. She did return to see him once but then terminated the relationship. Amy became increasingly depressed. She recalled feeling more dirty and evil than before. She retreated and rarely left home. She felt unfit to fulfill her responsibilities as a mother and experienced the physical fatigue of depression.

Amy became increasingly depressed and found her life unbearable. She told Bill she was leaving, that she was disgusting and dirty and shouldn't be raising children. She saw another male therapist, but when he touched her knee in what was apparently an innocent gesture, she became angry and refused to return.

She saw a television show regarding the abuse of clients by helping professionals. She wrote for and received additional information. She recalled bartering with God whether to tell Bill about her experiences with Mike. She resolved to tell him. After telling Bill about the sexual nature of the sessions with Mike, Amy attempted suicide for a third time. Again, she survived the attempt. Bill insisted she pursue litigation against Mike to prove the relationship was as she depicted it. They contacted an attorney and subsequently met to discuss and file a lawsuit.

Bill then took Amy to a hospital for inpatient care. The time Amy spent waiting in the hospital lobby became a turning point in her life. A man waiting in the lobby frightened her.

This idiot, this sick man, was sitting across from me staring at me. He was just openly staring at me. And, then he got up and moved closer to me. And that really bothered me, and I started becoming very afraid. There were no staff around, and I couldn't even see Bill. At that point, I remember thinking "it really doesn't matter." So I resolved myself to "I don't care, he can just come over here and do what he wants to." I remember that it was like being on a cliff, where you're either going to step off or turn around. I guess I decided to turn around a little bit.

When Bill returned with the admission papers for Amy to sign, she refused to stay. The physician and Bill discussed an emergency committal, but decided Amy could try being treated on an outpatient basis. She stayed with her parents and attended therapy sessions daily. She underwent another MMPI and evaluations, at her attorney's request, to ascertain her stability in pursuing the trial. At one point, she was diagnosed as bipolar and took lithium but later decided to discontinue it, on her own.

During the following spring, Amy decided to apply to a collegiate nursing program at a local college. She was initially turned away and told she was not capable of collegiate study. Amy persisted by writing placement exams to prove she was capable. The college later reconsidered when her placement scores exceeded those required. Amy then began college, a dream she had previously thought impossible. Amy busied herself with a full college course load and caring for her children, but tension between Bill and Amy was constant throughout the year. Amy had originally agreed to file the lawsuit against Mike to appease Bill, who wanted a vent for his anger and proof that Amy's version of the therapy sessions was true. Mike's defense attorneys claimed the suit was based on revenge; that Amy and Mike had become involved in a love affair, and when Mike refused to leave his wife, Amy retaliated with a lawsuit. Amy had convinced herself that the case would be settled out of court and that she would never have to actually testify. At one point during the year-long wait, negotiations to settle out of court were pursued. Bill asked for a lump sum of $30,000 to cover the cost of Amy's therapy, but Mike refused, claiming he did not have the money.

The trial date was set for fall, which caught Amy off guard. She was enrolled in nursing school and would have to request time away from her studies and clinical rotations to pursue the trial. She recalled fearing rejection from the nursing program if the faculty learned of her history. She contemplated dropping the charges; the thought of testifying terrified her anyway, but she then realized the trial had come to mean more to her. Pursuing the trial was no longer primarily for Bill's needs, but for her own; she wanted validation of her perceptions and victimization. Amy decided to pursue the trial and requested to be excused from her clinical duties.

The trial uncovered details of Amy's life that she would have preferred forgetting. She found her life was opened to examination, critique, and publication in the local newspapers.

> In court, this story's told about you and your life and things that have happened that really, 2 years before you had not even told your husband. And all of a sudden, everybody has access to it, the newspapers, the jury, the judge, the attorneys; all these people have such private and personal information about you. I hated that. I felt so violated by that, but I felt so much more violated by him.

Amy found the courtroom to be threatening. She recalled her side of the courtroom was bare, while Mike's side was full of supporters. Amy's family did not attend the trial, although they lived only 50 miles away. Two of her girlfriends did attend, and along with two total strangers, were the sole occupants of the prosecution's audience. During the trial, Amy wondered who the two strangers, a man and a woman, were; she assumed they were supporting Mike but were unable to find a vacant seat on his side of the courtroom. Mike's wife, secretary, clients, congregation, friends, and fellow deacons filled his side of the courtroom daily. Many community members, including his minister, testified in his defense.

Amy was fearful throughout the trial. Daily accounts of testimony were detailed in the local newspaper, which sensationalized the case. Threatening remarks were frequently made by the many people who believed in Mike and his capabilities as a counselor. They believed Amy and Bill were unjustly punishing Mike for Amy's situation. One evening, while sitting in their hotel room, a large object was hurled through their window. Subsequently, the attorneys moved the couple frequently in an attempt to maintain their security. Threatening phone calls persisted throughout the trial.

Throughout the trial, the defense attorneys strategized to blame Amy for Mike's behavior. Their relationship was publicized as "an affair gone bad." Depositions examined by me revealed accusations and the defense attorneys' referring to Amy as "a pretty little lady," which she recalled angered her immensely. He proceeded to refer to her by using this phrase repeatedly, which she perceived was an attempt to elicit a reaction from her. She recalls feeling the defense reinforced her sense of guilt by repeatedly focusing on her choice to continue seeing Mike after he began behaving sexually and argued that all Amy had to do was quit attending his sessions. The defense accusations took a toll on Amy's sense of self-esteem. She felt blamed for Mike's behavior.

Finally, the trial came to an end. Amy feared losing the case, recalling she felt the defense attorneys had painted Mike as a saint that Amy had tainted. However, the jury returned a guilty verdict and ordered Mike to pay twice the amount sought, close to half a million dollars. Amy and Bill were ecstatic while Mike's supporters became more hostile. When Bill and Amy tried to leave the courtroom, the man and woman who had been sitting on their side of the courtroom during the trial approached them. Amy felt certain they planned to hurt her and she froze. The man asked to shake her hand, and although she remembered being sensitive to touch, she extended her hand to him. He introduced himself as a visiting relative of a jury member and expressed his respect for her. Next, the woman approached her and asked to embrace Amy. Amy agreed and remembered the embrace as "genuine, like hugging yourself." Amy asked the woman if she had been abused by a therapist, and she indicated she had but quickly left before Amy could inquire if the abuse had been inflicted by Mike.

Amy would return to testify against Mike a second time, in a suit brought by another client he sexually abused. Learning that Mike had abused other clients confirmed Amy's belief that pursuing the suit had been worthwhile. In the subsequent suit a settlement was reached before the victim ever testified.

Mike's insurance company refused to pay the court award, and Mike hid his assets by transferring all of his property to his father. Mike's license was revoked by the licensing board. Bill and Amy filed an appeal and maintained faith that the jury's intentions would materialize. Amy returned to school and attacked her studies with diligence. She spent most of her time studying or involved in schoolwork. She was a class officer and graduated with highest honors.

Following graduation, Amy began work in a local hospital on a full-time basis. Amy and Bill's marital relationship stabilized following the trial. The family resumed a less stressful existence. The following spring, the couple learned their appeal had been denied by the local court. The attorney suggested appealing to the district court, which they pursued. The family continued to maintain hope of receiving the jury's award. Later in the year, Amy learned their appeal had been denied in district court. The couple was left with monumental attorney and psychotherapy fees, both of which were to be paid by Mike according to the jury. Amy maintains that, although the family has been denied the monetary award, she still feels rewarded.

I know I would not be functioning as well now, and my life would be very different had there been a different decision retained from the jury. I was so ready to blame myself, and I had such a sense of responsibility that I couldn't forgive myself. If they had said, "this is your doing; this is your fault," I don't think I could have withstood it.

Amy agreed to participate in this study a few years after losing the court appeal. She participated in interviews for 4 months, followed by assisting in the validation of content analysis for 5 months. She hopes sharing her experiences will be helpful to others and talks of things that had been helpful to her, like the support of others. Amy and Bill have remained together, despite experiencing emotional turmoil. His support has contributed to her perception of herself as valuable.

Amy believes the stress of the trial ultimately strengthened her relationship with Bill, although initially it seemed certain the trial would destroy their marriage. Attorneys had advised Amy to consider the consequences of losing her husband and children before proceeding with the trial. She recalled at the time thinking she would lose her family anyway, so she thought she had nothing to lose. She recalls Bill's brother encouraging him to leave her, but he decided to stay.

One of the rewarding things about the whole thing, I'll just call it the culmination, emerging with an affirmation. We've been through so much, and there's been recoil and re-evaluation of "is it worth it?" To find that he stood by me; I expected him, and I was told that he would probably walk, that when this was revealed to him that I shouldn't expect him to stay.

She is trying to make up for lost time with her children. Both her interactions with her children and her descriptions of them clearly illustrate her appreciation of her children. Both are all-American boys. They talk openly of things some parents avoid, such as sex. Amy recalled fearing the oldest would grow up hating her because she was so unpredictable when he was young, but that was not the case. Amy recognizes the relationship she has with her sons as a gift to be appreciated.

Amy's belief in a higher power has aided her. She believes her life has been guided and protected and that God has taken care of her. On several occasions, she has made choices that could have exacerbated her situation but instead improved the circumstances.

She recalled attending college as providing an avenue for channeling her energy and anger.

I still believe in a thousand ways it saved my sanity, more than therapy. It gave me a focus and fulfilled my old goals. It was a goal I had control over cause I had no way of controlling the trial. It was a bridge that got me over all that ugliness; when I saw that I could succeed at nursing, 'cause nursing is the symbol of goodness and caring directed outwardly for the benefit of others.

She also reported a persistent feeling that she was an evil person and a quote from a play, in which an ugly ostracized child is accepted, she found helpful.

It just summed it up for me. I knew everything about me was hideous and ugly and repulsive, but I was gonna have to learn to kiss it and to like it and to live with it because I couldn't escape it any more. And that's what it came down to. With the trial and everything, that's still what it came down to, learning to accept who I am and learning to love it and realizing that this is who I am.

Amy's beliefs regarding her personal and sexual rights have changed considerably. As a child she was socialized to expect abuse from family members and raised in a culture in which sexual abuse of women and children was the norm. She has learned and asserts her rights to be treated with respect yet still struggles with cognitive dissonance at times.

DISCUSSION

This study examined the lived experience of incestuous abuse and subsequent sexual exploitation by a helping professional. Data collected by the use of the life history technique were examined, and themes identified were validated by the respondent. The prevalence of each of the 23 themes identified: anger, control, loss, betrayal, guilt, magical thinking, powerlessness, rescuing others, need to belong, retreat, fantasy, unreasonable expectations, cultural sanctions, diffuse boundaries, risk-taking, ambivalence, affirmation of value, tenacity, assertion, insight, acceptance, appreciation, and hope were correlated with the four developmental stages of childhood, adolescence, young adulthood, and adulthood. Owing to the page limitations of this chapter, the extended discussion is not repeated here. Anger, control, and affirmation of value emerged as consistent themes and were therefore identified as central. Amy validated the consistent presence of these three themes throughout her life. Amy also recognized the theme of acceptance as being key to her resolution of internal conflicts, so it was included as a central theme of her life. The remaining 19 themes may be viewed as subcomponents, contributors, or outcomes of the four central themes and are therefore viewed as secondary.

The cultural sanctions that condoned abuse and devaluation of women and children provided a milieu beyond Amy's control. Unreasonable expectations, such as holding children responsible for avoiding abuse, coupled with confused boundaries and roles, left Amy anxious, uncertain, and with a feeling of being ineffectual or powerless. Fantasy and magical thinking provided cognitive means of exerting control. Amy pursued a career in which she could rescue others to feel competent and powerful. Ambivalence was a common emotion for Amy, as she feared her choices might lead to failure. She strived to control the outcome of her choices. Her need to belong led her to struggle for the acceptance of others and search for validation of her worth. Thus, the issue of control emerges from several sources: (a) others exerting control over Amy; (b) Amy exerting control over others; and (c) Amy's struggle to control her emotions, behavior, and relationships. When others control Amy, through abuse, manipulation, or withholding information, she feels powerless and angry. Exerting control reduces feelings of powerlessness and provides a sense of security, predictability, and comfort for Amy. The primary themes of anger and control are interrelated to the secondary themes cited.

Throughout her life, others have given Amy messages affirming her value and importance. These messages were provided by her grandmother, her peers, a junior high school teacher, health care providers, her husband, therapists, and by Amy herself. The messages may have been influential in enabling Amy to persevere and believe in herself.

Amy also recognized the concept of acceptance as key to her present level of functioning. She examined those undesirable and seemingly intolerable components of her life and gradually accepted and embraced them as undeniably hers. Through accepting herself unconditionally, she became more self-trusting, confident, assertive, and also more accepting of others.

In examining the sequencing of theme emergence, Amy recognized the trial as a turning point in her life. The jury's verdict validated her perception of her abuse and enabled her to accept her past without guilt. Those themes, which only emerged or became stronger after the trial, namely, assertion, insight, appreciation, and hope, may be viewed as outcomes of Amy's self-acceptance. Those themes more prevalent prior to the trial may be subcomponents of the themes of anger and control. The persistent theme of affirmation of value may have exerted a mediating effect, enabling Amy to endure abuses and accept her anger and control issues.

The themes of risk-taking and tenacity seem to be personal attributes of Amy but may also be related to the themes of anger and control. In review of Amy's life, the primary and secondary themes, and the changes she has experienced, the following propositions are posited: (a) through accepting her anger and control issues, Amy was able to integrate her abusive experiences into her life without them consuming her existence; (b) messages that affirmed her value fostered Amy's self-acceptance; and (c) Amy's self-acceptance enabled her to channel her energies into productive avenues instead of self-destructive behaviors.

SUMMARY

In summary, the life experiences of the respondent were expressed through 23 themes identified by me and validated by the respondent. Nineteen themes were classified as secondary, relating to the primary themes of anger, control, acceptance, and affirmation. A typology, correlating the 19 secondary themes with Amy's developmental phases, revealed the prevalence of each theme throughout the respondent's life. The prevalence of each theme was examined within the context of the critical incidents of each developmental level. Three propositions that attempt to explain the integration of the respondent's experiences were generated. A conceptual model was devised to illustrate the uniqueness of the respondent's life and the propositions proposed.

Concepts Related to Literature

Four themes were central to the respondent's experiences, and the remaining 19 themes were classified as secondary. A conceptual model was developed to illustrate the uniqueness of Amy's experience. Propositional statements were posed and validated by the respondent as potential explanations of her experience. The findings of this study do not fully support nor refute the review of research. Amy did report experiencing many of the symptoms identified as immediate and lasting effects of incestuous abuse, as well as those reported in clients experiencing therapist sexual exploitation. Amy's experience also reflects themes that have thus far been omitted from the research literature.

Amy reported being aggressive and anxious to please others as a child, traits that Conte and Schuerman (1988) reported. Amy characterized her adolescence as consumed with depression, alcohol and drug use, and social isolation, traits which were reported in the Conte and Schuerman (1988); Herman and Hirschman (1981), and Anderson and colleagues (1981) samples. Amy also reported leaving home during adolescence and suspicion of men, a finding reported in the Miesleman (1978) samples.

Brunngraber's (1986) findings most closely resemble Amy's experiences. Amy reported experiencing suppressed emotion, social isolation, negative self-image, powerlessness, fear of physical contact with men, and few female friends, as reported in the Brunngraber sample. Some factors identified in the Brunngraber sample, reported as being more subtle influences in her life, include displeasure with her physical appearance, persistent "female trouble," and vacillating between promiscuity and celibacy. Amy's experience also reflects many of the characteristics identified in the research regarding lasting effects of incestuous abuse. Amy's persistent depression was also noted in the Sedney and Brooks (1984), Briere and Runtz (1986), and Peters (1988) samples. Amy's three suicide attempts validate the suicidality reported by Sedney and Brooks (1984) and Goodwin (1989).

The isolation, anger, betrayal, sadness, loss, powerlessness, and emotional control reported in the Edwards and Donaldson (1989) sample were consistent with Amy's experience. Amy's father was physically abusive, her mother passive and distant, and she was socialized into maternal duties at the age of 13.

Furthermore, several of the lasting effects noted by Brunngraber (1986) were also reported by Amy, namely, feeling different from others, insecurity, drug and alcohol use, guilt, distrust of men, and menstrual difficulties.

The positive outcomes noted by Amy can be compared with the findings of Brunngraber (1986), the sole researcher to report any positive outcomes of incestuous abuse. Like the Brunngraber sample, Amy expressed increased sensitivity toward others, increased self-reliance, insight, and understanding through self-examination and reflection. But unlike the Brunngraber sample, Amy has not become closer to her family members. Amy's family did not support her in her time of need, a factor identified as unifying the families of the Brunngraber sample.

As for the limited research in the area of sexual exploitation by therapists, Amy's experience was consistent with some of the symptoms reported by the Bouhoutsos, Holroyd, Lerman, Fover, and Greenberg (1983) sample. Amy experienced mistrust of men, marital difficulties, and mistrust of therapists. However, each of these traits was reported by Amy prior to Mike's abuse, so a linear relationship cannot be assumed. Like the Bouhoutsos and colleagues (1983) and Vinson (1984) samples, Amy reported believing the primary issues that brought her to therapy in the first place worsened as a result of neglect and became complicated by a therapist's sexual abuse. Like the Pope and Bouhoutsos (1986) sample, Amy reported prolonged emotional upheaval, powerlessness, and feeling she had become the defendant as a result of pursuing legal recourse for her abuse.

Although there are several areas of agreement between Amy's experiences and the effects reported in the research, total congruence does not exist. Many of the symptoms noted in the literature review were not reported by Amy. Thus, the fact that Amy's experience is consistent with some of the issues identified in the research cannot serve to validate or refute the findings of neither the previous nor of this work. It should be remembered that this research was not intended to produce generalizable results but to enhance understanding and insight through examination of the experience as it was lived by the person who had the experience .

As few of the themes that connote strengths, healthy attributes, or positive outcomes were found in the review of research, these warrant additional attention. The themes of hope, appreciation, acceptance, insight, assertion, tenacity, affirmation of value, and risk-taking have thus far eluded researchers. Amy's experiences with each of these health-oriented themes will be briefly examined. Amy's hope springs from an internal motivation for a better life. Prior to the incident in the hospital lobby, she had searched for reasons or justification for hope in her external environment. She had found increasingly sparse external evidence that her hopes would be realized. Instead of giving up, Amy looked inside for the strength to persevere. She quoted an excerpt from a play in which a character realizes that depending on external sources of hope is risky, and the only reliable source must come from within. Through self-reflection, she has gained considerable insight into her behavior and emotions. Amy learned the techniques of analyzing emotions and behaviors in therapy and found she felt such control and power from the use of these techniques that they have become an obsession. She hopes to become less obsessed with gaining understanding of all of her emotions and behavior in the future.

Through repeated self-examination and analysis of the abusive experiences of her life, and reading of other's experiences, Amy gained a sense of relativity. She views her experiences within the context of those experienced by others. Increased media coverage and publication of abusive cases has heightened her awareness of the global nature of sexual abuse. As painful as her abuses were, she expressed appreciation that they had not been worse. Amy appreciates her husband and children. Once convinced that she would lose her husband, her children, and her sanity, Amy appreciates routines that others may perceive monotonous. She appreciates the stability of owning a home after 11 moves prior to, and 8 more moves during, her marriage. She expressed gratitude for the daily gifts many take for granted.

Amy's self-reliance emerged from a realization that she is the only person she can always rely on, a discovery made in the lobby of a psychiatric hospital. Her assertion has emerged from gaining self-acceptance and mitigating the intensity of her anger through ventilation. Through therapy, Amy confronted the unreasonable expectations she held and began accepting herself unconditionally. Amy's risk-taking behaviors are based on trust. Theoretically, people will not risk unless they trust that the outcome will outweigh the risk involved. The attribute of trust has influenced her behavior, decisions, and tenacity, a theme that is apparent throughout Amy's life. Her persistence and refusal to give up are positive attributes.

Implications

Implications of this research lie in the 23 themes identified and are both clinical and theoretical in nature. Clinical implications are classified into primary, secondary, and tertiary prevention. Theoretical implications follow the clinical implication discussion.

Clinical Implications

Primary prevention is concerned with measures that may prevent abuse from occurring. A great deal of research has focused on educational programs that instruct children in sexual rights, psychological self-defense, and techniques to avoid abusive situations. These programs are usually geared toward the school-aged child, excluding those possibly most vulnerable, the younger child. Furthermore, these programs focus on teaching the child strategies, implying the child is capable of preventing sexual abuse. Nonetheless, had Amy received any exposure to prevention strategies or sexual rights, she may have responded differently to both the farmhand's molestation and the bus rape. Parents need education regarding the vulnerability of their children, even within their immediate family. Protective strategies are needed, including strategies to intervene with cultural sanctioning and acceptance of abuse of children. Amy's parents socialized her into the abusive culture they had always known. Had her parents been exposed to information regarding cultural contributors to vulnerability and holding adults, especially offenders, accountable for their behavior, they may have been better prepared to protect Amy and institute sanctions against intrafamilial offenders.

Open communication and increased involvement between parents and children is imperative. Amy recalled both of her parents as distant and only attending to her when her behavior inconvenienced them. Had she felt they were interested in her, she may have disclosed her abuses to them. However, when Amy tried to tell her parents of her suicidal impulses, her father encouraged her to act on them. Nurses play an integral role in the assessment of family needs and communication patterns and must recognize and use opportunities to address the psychosocial health and well-being of family members in their clinical practice.

Adaptive coping skills are essential to the mental health of everyone but are of particular importance to those who experience sexual abuse. Anticipatory guidance such as role playing potential situations may prepare both children and parents for abuse. Had Amy felt comfortable with her right to say "No" to adults, she may have responded differently to the farmhand and her Uncle Sam. Parents must anticipate their child's vulnerability for abuse to prepare themselves psychologically and provide essential support to the child. In addition to teaching and role modeling coping skills and anticipatory guidance, nurses must practice the elements of crisis intervention when abuse occurs. The three components of crisis intervention, the individual's perception of the event, coping skills, and support systems, provide a framework for nursing assessment, intervention, and evaluation. Nurses must be sensitive to the needs of victims. When Amy presented to the emergency room with an overdose of codeine at age 16, a nurse may have been instrumental in helping Amy express herself verbally, instead of internalizing her emotions.

In the area of sexual exploitation by a helping professional, primary prevention measures include disclosure of ethical codes of conduct and increased awareness of sexual misconduct within the helping professions. As clients are required to share complete history and personal data forms prior to being assessed by a therapist, this seems an appropriate source for advising clients about sexual misconduct. Information regarding ethical and unethical practices, how to respond to sexual contact, and how to report such behavior could be included in the client's consent to treatment document. If Amy had been exposed to information regarding unethical conduct prior to being treated by Mike, she may have responded very differently to his advances. The curricula of those in the helping professions must address the issue of sexual misconduct to heighten awareness among those providing therapy. Licensing and regulating boards should be accountable for close scrutiny of allegations of unethical conduct by therapists.

Secondary prevention strategies are those intended to reduce the prevalence of illness. Therapists working with those who have experienced incestuous abuse must possess specific knowledge and skills regarding the nature of incest and therapist sexual exploitation if successful outcomes are to be realized. Amy expressed both displeasure and disappointment with most of the nine therapists from whom she sought help. Even though Amy recognized that she was seeking relief, she also felt that most of the therapists had no appreciation for her particular issues. Had Amy seen a therapist skilled in dealing with the dynamics of incestuous abuse, she may have experienced less turmoil, incurred fewer expenses and evaluations, and emerged even healthier than she managed on her own. Incest, as a sociocultural problem, must be included in the education of all in the helping professions in an effort to enhance prompt case recognition. Yet, once cases are recognized, skilled treatment relies on a body of specified knowledge and experience and should be available to those who seek professional assistance. Disciplines that educate therapists should develop sexual abuse subspecialty curricula.

Peer review of therapeutic strategies and ethical codes of behavior is also indicated. Even the standard use of supervision did not impede Mike's abuse of Amy; he simply neglected to tell his supervisor of their sessions. All therapists, including supervisors, need to be cognizant and sensitive to the issues of ethical codes of conduct. The dynamic of transference influenced Amy's receptivity to Mike's advances and thus should be examined as potentially influential in each client–therapist relationship. In Amy's situation, Mike was a popular counselor who enjoyed a community and religious following, which may have fostered others' unquestioning faith. This skewed cultural milieu influenced Amy's transference and vulnerability to his advances.

Given the variables Amy identified as being helpful to her, therapists may wish to consider addressing the following issues with clients who have been incestuously abused and sexually exploited by a therapist. The client's strengths are to be evaluated and reinforced. Amy's strengths of tenacity, affirmation of value, acceptance, insight, and assertion were attributes she used to reframe her experiences and integrate them into her life. Spouses and family members may require therapeutic attention to address their own concerns and to learn supportive measures to affirm the client's sense of value and importance. Bill may have been better prepared to support Amy had he understood her behavior and the dynamics that enabled Mike to abuse her under the guise of therapy. Bill could have also benefited from assistance in ventilating his anger. Clear consistent messages regarding the offender's responsibility for his behavior may have helped relieve Amy's sense of guilt.

The concepts of hope, insight, assertion, affirmation of value, and power appear to have been key to therapeutic healing for Amy. These phenomena warrant examination by the therapeutic community. Means of instilling, reinforcing, or activating these phenomena should be examined, and therapeutic strategies devised and tested. To prevent or counteract powerlessness, sources of power should be identified and mobilized. The concept of empowerment holds promise in the development of therapeutic interventions.

Teaching clients techniques of analyzing behavioral patterns, emotional responses, and interactions with others may provide them with a sense of control and power. Amy relied on these techniques, as they helped her label emotions and understand her own behavior and that of others. This understanding helped her feel more in control, less anxious, and more capable, or powerful. Confronting unrealistic expectations, sexual myths, and cultural sanctions aided Amy in creating change through self-reflection. Techniques to facilitate self-understanding and insight may encourage self-acceptance.

Therapeutic strategies that foster the channeling of anger into productive avenues were helpful to Amy. Incest victims may have intense anger that needs ventilation. Uncontrolled expression can lead to self-destructive behavior, suicide, or homicide. Identifying challenges the client is interested in and supporting his or her pursuit of goals was a therapeutic strategy that Amy recognized as helpful and that led to her graduation from college.

Methods of fostering acceptance of things beyond the client's control warrant attention. Amy began to view her situation within the context of others through the use of bibliotherapy, reading about others' abusive experiences, and attending to media coverage of abuse cases. Exposure to others' experiences provided validation, a perspective of relativity, and appreciation for Amy. Group therapy, which also provides the experience of universality, may also facilitate acceptance.

Therapists must consider that the dynamic of resistance is not the sole reason clients leave therapy; Amy was, for instance, ventilating her anger toward therapists through exercising control and power. Changing therapists was therapeutic for Amy. Historically, the literature has reflected the belief that the therapeutic relationship, in particular the working phase of the relationship, is contingent on the development of trust. Frequent rejection of therapists would seem to impair the development of trust. Yet, Amy was so mistrustful of therapists following her experiences with Mike that developing trust may have been an unrealistic goal.

Rejection provided a means of ventilating anger through retaliation and gave Amy a sense of power and control, both of which were healthy. For those abused by a therapist, the therapeutic value of pursuing legal recourse warrants attention. The process is obviously stressful to the plaintiff and the potential benefits must be weighed against the risks of the offender being exonerated. Although the validation of a jury trial provided unsurpassed therapeutic value to Amy, she also recognized her life would be very different had Mike been found innocent. Careful preparation for questioning and testimony enabled Amy to withstand the defense interrogation.

Therapeutic support throughout the trial proceedings was essential for both Amy and Bill. Assistive programs for the plaintiffs and their families could be funded through offender fees levied at the time the verdict is entered. Automatic salary garnishment seems necessary to ensure payment of the plaintiff's attorney and therapy fees as well as any award granted by the jury.

Salary garnishment would rectify the complexities created when a liability insurance company refuses to pay a claim and attorneys lose interest, owing to their inability to recover their fee. If found guilty, the liability for attorney and therapy fees should automatically be placed on the offender to prevent a reoccurrence of Amy's situation; she and Bill faced six-digit debt for attorney and therapist fees.

Tertiary prevention focuses on ongoing support. As previously mentioned, group support may be helpful. Bibliotherapy and attention to media coverage may provide a gradual sense of acceptance and relativity. Maintaining a diary, writing an autobiography, or participating in a life history review may offer the opportunity to evaluate and integrate lived experiences. Life review provided Amy with a sense of closure, which she believed necessary to proceeding forward with a sense of closure of her past.

Like incest, the sexual abuse of clients by therapists may be more prevalent than suspected. As offenders, therapists must address the issues and dynamics that led to such behavior if change can ever occur. Owing to the power differential that is characteristic of the therapy environment, therapists who offend must not be allowed to continue practicing.

Theoretical Implications

Thus far, the theoretical literature has focused on preconditions to abuse and why societies tolerate abuse rather than on describing the experience and prescribing successful resolutions. Theories that depict the experience will provide insight for clients and therapists alike. Theories that prescribe means of facilitating acceptance and healthy resolution are essential to the therapeutic functions of practice-oriented disciplines such as nursing.

Inductive strategies should begin with identification of the phenomena of interest such as the central themes identified in this study. Examination of the lives of others who have experienced incestuous abuse and sexual exploitation by a therapist is indicated to discover additional themes. Purposive sampling techniques should be employed to ensure a heterogeneous sample. Heterogeneous samples will provide a vast array of realities, theme variability, and a broad pool of data for theory development.

Once identified, attributes and characteristics of the phenomena of interest must be discerned. Conceptual analysis of the central themes isolated in this study, and themes isolated from future studies, would aid in concept recognition, measurement, and the development of therapeutic strategies. Themes identified must be measured in a wide variety of situations, again to ensure variability of results. Analysis of the resulting data will reveal any systematic patterns among the phenomena. Working hypotheses must then be generated and tested through respondent reviews. Patterns are then refined and expressed in the form of theoretical statements. Studies can then be devised to test the adequacy and validity of the theoretical statements. If empirical findings fail to support the theoretical statement, and the research design is unflawed, the theoretical statement must be altered to reflect reality and retested. Subsequently, each statement is tested to refine and strengthen the theory.

This study represents the first case in the development of a descriptive theory of the lived experience of incest and sexual exploitation by a therapist. In addition to describing the experience, central themes were isolated. The data obtained also provided insight into facilitative and inhibitory factors experienced by Amy during her process of resolution. Thus, factors were isolated and related to an outcome. Propositions were generated, validated as plausible by the respondent, and offered for subsequent testing and refinement. These steps must be replicated before any specific relationship between themes and a desirable outcome can be explicated, enabling the development of factor-relating and situation-relating level theory. Situation-producing theory, which depicts strategies to facilitate client acceptance and resolution, is the ultimate goal.

In summary, implications for clinical practice were proposed in the areas of primary, secondary, and tertiary prevention. Theoretical implications lie in the dearth of theory in the area. As the current status of theory development in the area of incest is inadequate, suggestions were made for theory development. The experience of incest and sexual exploitation by a therapist remains unknown. This study represents the first of many steps needed to develop factor-isolating theory that answers the question, "What is the experience?" Factor-relating theory must then be developed to address the relationships among factors. Desirable outcomes, such as in Amy's case, integration and resolution of her abusive experiences and issues, must be identified, described, measured, and related to other factors. Factors that facilitate and inhibit healthy resolution must then be identified. Lastly, therapeutic strategies must be developed to foster resolution of the experience. Theory development at all levels is needed to understand the experience and respond knowledgeably and therapeutically to it.

Recommendations

The following are recommendations for future theory-generating and theory-testing research, in order of priority.

Theory Generation

1. Replication of this study, utilizing heterogeneous respondents, is essential to ascertain the lived experience of incest and sexual exploitation by a therapist. Heterogeneous respondents will provide a rich data source of multiple realities, thereby enhancing understanding of the lived experience from the emic perspective. Questions that need further clarification include, What is the experience?, What are the healthy attributes of the respondent?, What is considered a desirable outcome of the experience?, How can incest and sexual exploitation by a therapist be survived? These questions must be answered for the development of factor-isolating level theories.
2. Once isolated, themes that represent the experience must be closely examined, their qualities and characteristics identified, and operational definitions constructed. Questions that remain unanswered include, What is the experience of each of the themes identified as central? For example, What is the experience of anger? Of control? Of acceptance? Of affirmation of value? Of resolution? What are the characteristics of messages that affirm value?
3. Relationships among themes must be discerned and posited in the form of plausible propositions. Propositions are then to be tested and refined into theoretical statements that link themes. Questions to be addressed include, What is the relationship between themes and outcomes?, What facilitated resolution of the experience?, What inhibited resolution?, How can clinicians facilitate resolution? These questions must be answered for the development of factor-relating, situation-relating, and situation-producing level theory.

Theory Testing

1. Valid tools must be developed to measure the presence and intensity of each of the themes. Tools are essential for theme recognition in clients.
2. Mixed design studies are indicated, using tools to quantify and interviewing to qualify the themes, outcomes, and experiences.
3. The theoretical statement of each theory developed must be empirically tested. If supported, other statements must be tested to determine the practice limitations of the theory. If a statement is not supported by reality, it must be refined and retested. This step will lead to the development of valid theories, which are essential for theory-guided practice.
4. Therapeutic strategies, posited by situation-producing theory, must be tested with clinical samples and refined for the development of specific interventions.

REFERENCES

Anderson, S., Bach, C., & Griffith, C. (1981). *Psychosocial sequelae in intrafamilial victims of sexual assault and abuse.* Paper presented at the Third International Conference on Child Abuse and Neglect. Amsterdam, the Netherlands.

Black, H. C. (1979). *Black's law dictionary* (5th ed.). St. Paul, MN: West.

Bouhoutsos, J., Holroyd, J., Lerman, H., Fover, B., & Greenberg, M. (1983). Sexual intimacy between psychotherapists and patients. *Professional Psychologist, 14*(2), 185–196.

Briere, J., & Runtz, M. (1986). Suicidal thoughts and behavior in sexual abuse survivors. *Canadian Journal of Behavioral Science, 18,* 413–423.

Browne, S., & Finkelhor, D. (1986). The impact of child sexual abuse: A review of the research. *Psychological Bulletin, 99,* 66–77.

Brunngraber, L. S. (1986). Father-daughter incest: Immediate and long-term effects of sexual abuse. *Advances in Nursing Science, 4,* 15–35.

Burgess, A. W., Groth, A. N., Holstrom, L. L., & Sgroi, S. (Ed.). (1978). *Sexual assault of children and adolescents.* Lexington, MA: Lexington Books.

Burgess, A. W., & Hartman, C. R. (Eds.). (1986). *Sexual exploitation of patients by health professionals.* New York, NY: Praeger.

Burns, N. (1989). Standards for qualitative research. *Nursing Science Quarterly, 1*(1), 44–52.

Cambell, J., & Humphreys, J. (1984). *Nursing care of victims of family violence.* Reston, VA: Reston Publishing.

Chenitz, W. C., & Swanson, J. M. (1986). *From practice to grounded theory: Qualitative research in nursing.* Menlo Park, CA: Addison-Wesley.

Constantine, L. (1980). Effects of early sexual experience: A review and synthesis of research. In L. Constantine & F. M. Martinson (Eds.), *Children and sex* (pp. 114–132). Boston, MA: Little, Brown, and Company.

Conte, J. R., & Schuerman, J. R. (1988). The effects of sexual abuse on children: A multidimensional view. In G. E. Wyatt & G. J. Powell (Eds.), *Lasting effects of child sexual abuse* (pp. 157–170). Beverly Hills, CA: Sage.

Courtois, C. A. (1988). *Healing the incest wound: Adult survivors in therapy.* New York, NY: Norton.

Crewdson, J. (1988). *By silence betrayed: Sexual abuse of children in America.* New York, NY: Harper and Row.

de Chesnay, M. (1985). Father-daughter incest: An overview. *Behavioral Sciences and the Law, 4*(4), 391–402.

Derosia, H., Hamilton, J., Morrison, E., & Strauss, M. (1987). More on psychiatrist-patient sexual contact. *American Journal of Psychiatry, 144,* 688–689.

Dobbert, M. C. (1982). *Ethnographic research.* New York, NY: Praeger.

Donaldson, N. E. (1987). The phenmenological method: Qualitatively advancing nursing science. In S. R. Gartner (Ed.), *Nursing science methods: A reader* (pp. 88–92). San Francisco: Regents, University of California.

Edwards, P. W., & Donaldson, M. A. (1989). Assessment of symptoms in adult survivors of incest: A factor analytic study of the Responses to Childhood Incest Questionnaire. *Child Abuse and Neglect, 13,* 101–110.

Field, P. A., & Morse, J. M. (1985). *Nursing research: The application of qualitative approaches.* Rockville, MD: Aspen.

Finkelhor, D. (1979). What's wrong with sex between adults and children? *American Journal of Orthopsychiatry, 49,* 692–697.

Finkelhor, D. (1984). *Child sexual abuse: New research and theory.* New York, NY: The Free Press.

Finkelhor, D. (1986). *A sourcebook on child sexual abuse.* Newbury Park, CA: Sage.

Finkelhor, D. (1987). The sexual abuse of children: Current research reviewed. *Psychiatric Annals, 17*(4), 233–241.

Forward, S., & Buck, C. (1978). *Betrayal of innocence: Incest and its devastation.* New York, NY: Penguin Books.

Friedrich, W. N. (1988). Behavior problems in sexually abused children: An adaptational perspective. In G. Wyatt & G. Powell (Eds.), *The lasting effects of child sexual abuse* (pp. 171–191). Newbury Park, CA: Sage.

Friedrich, W. N., Urquiza, A. J., & Beilke, R. (1986). Behavioral problems in sexually abused children. *Journal of Pediatric Psychology, 11*(2), 47–57.

Gartrell, H., Herman, J. L., & Olarte, S. (1986). Psychiatrist-patient sexual contact: Results of a national survey, I: Prevalence. *American Journal of Psychiatry, 143,* 1126–1131.

Goldman, R. L., & Wheeler, V. R. (1986). *The sexual abuse of children and youth: Silent shame.* Danville, IL: Interstate.

Goochman, D. S. (Ed.). (1988). *Health behavior: Emerging research perspectives.* New York, NY: Plenum Press.

Goodwin, J. (Ed.). (1989). *Sexual abuse: Incest victims and their families* (2nd ed.). Chicago: Year Book.

Grando, R. (1983). Incest: Understanding the dynamics and problems. *The Counseling Interviewer, 1*(12), 32–35.

Gruber, K., & Jones, R. (1983). Identifying determinants of risk of sexual victimization of youth. *Child Abuse and Neglect, 1*(2), 17–24.

Haugaard, J., & Reppucci, N. (1988). *The sexual abuse of children*. San Francisco: Jossey-Bass.

Henderson, J. (1983). Is incest harmful? *Canadian Journal of Psychiatry, 28*, 34–39.

Herman, J., & Hirschman, L. (1981). *Father-daughter incest*. Cambridge, MA: Harvard University Press.

Holroyd, J., & Brodsky, A. (1977). Psychologists' attitudes and practices regarding erotic and non-erotic contact with patients. *American Psychologist, 32*, 843–849.

Jacobsen, J. J. (1986). *Psychiatric sequelae of child abuse*. Springfield, IL: Charles C. Thomas.

Janeway, E. (1981, November). Incest: A national look at the oldest taboo. *Ms. Magazine*, 61–64.

Justice, B., & Justice, R. (1979). *The broken taboo: Sex in the family*. New York, NY: Human Sciences Press.

Kinsey, A. C., Pomeroy, W. B., Martin, C. E., & Gebhard, P. H. (1953). *Sexual behavior in the human female*. Philadelphia, PA: W. B. Saunders.

Kluft, R. P. (1989). Incest and subsequent re-victimization: The sitting duck syndrome. In R. P. Kluft (Ed.), *Incest-related syndromes of adult psychopathology*. Washington, DC: American Psychiatric Press.

Koch, M. (1980). Sexual abuse of children. *Adolescence, 15*, 643–648.

Landis, J. (1956). Experiences of 500 children with adult sexual deviants. *Psychiatric Quarterly Supplement, 30*, 91–109.

Langness, L. L., & Frank, G. (1981). *Lives: An anthropological approach to biography*. Novato, CA: Handler and Sharp.

Leininger, M. M. (Ed.). (1985). *Qualitative research methods in nursing*. New York, NY: Grune and Stratton.

Lincoln, Y. S., & Guba, E. (1985). *Naturalistic inquiry*. Beverly Hills, CA: Sage.

Miesleman, K. (1978). *Incest: A psychological study of causes and effects with treatment recommendations*. San Francisco: Jossey-Bass.

Miles, M. B., & Huberman, A. M. (1984). *Qualitative data analysis: A sourcebook of new methods*. Beverly Hills, CA: Sage.

National Center for the Prevention of Child Abuse and Neglect. (1981). Study findings: National study of the incidence and severity of child abuse and neglect. DHHS Publication (HDS) 81-30325. Washington, DC: US Government Printing Office.

Peters, S. D. (1988). Child sexual abuse and later psychological problems. In G. E. Wyatt & G. J. Powell (Eds.), *Lasting effects of child sexual abuse* (pp. 119–134). Beverly Hills, CA: Sage.

Plasil, E. (1985). *Therapist*. New York, NY: St. Martin's Press.

Pope, K. S., & Bouhoutsos, J. C. (1986). *Sexual intimacy between therapists and patients*. New York, NY: Praeger.

Pope, K. S., Keith-Spiegel, P. C., & Tabachnik, B. G. (1986). Sexual attraction to clients: The human therapist and (sometimes) inhuman training system. *American Psychologist, 41*, 147–158.

Ray, M. A. (1985). A philosophical method to study nursing phenomena. In M. M. Leininger (Ed.), *Qualitative research methods in nursing* (pp. 81–92). New York, NY: Grune and Stratton.

Robinson, L.(1982). Nursing therapy of an incest victim. *Issues in Mental Health Nursing, 4*, 331–342.

Russell, D. (1983). The incidence and prevalence of intrafamilial and extrafamilial sexual abuse of female children. *Child Abuse and Neglect, 1*(2), 133–146.

Russell, D. (1984). The prevalence and seriousness of incestuous abuse: Stepfathers vs. biological fathers. *Child Abuse and Neglect, 8*(1), 15–22.

Russell, D. (1986). *The secret trauma: Incest in the lives of girls and women.* New York, NY: Basic Books.

Sedney, M. A., & Brooks, B. (1984). Factors associated with a history of childhood sexual experience in a nonclinical female population. *Journal of American Academy of Child Psychiatry, 23*(3), 215–218.

Sgroi, S. (1988). *Vulnerable populations: Evaluation and treatment of sexually abused children and adult survivors.* Lexington, MA: Lexington Books.

Vander Mey, B. J., & Neff, R. L. (1982). Adult-child incest: A review of research and treatment. *Adolescence, 17*(4), 717–735.

Vander Mey, B. J., & Neff, R. L. (1986). *Incest as child abuse: Research and application.* New York, NY: Praeger.

Vinson, J. S. (1984). *Sexual contact with psychotherapists: A study of clients reactions and complaint procedures.* Unpublished doctoral dissertation, California School of Professional Psychology.

Walker, E., & Young, T. A. (1986). *A killing cure.* New York, NY: Henry Holt.

Watson, L. C., & Watson-Franke, M. B. (1985). *Interpreting life histories: An anthropological inquiry.* New Brunswick, NJ: Rutgers University Press.

Wyatt, G. E., & Peters, S. O. (1986). Issues in the definition of child sexual abuse in prevalence research. *Child Abuse and Neglect, 10*(3), 231–240.

Wyatt, G. E., & Powell, G. J. (Eds.). (1988). *Lasting effects of child sexual abuse.* Newbury Park, CA: Sage.

Chapter Five

Whistleblowing as Self-Reported Disclosure by Incest Survivors

Edwina Skiba-King

*I*n the early 1960s, a new phenomenon emerged in large bureaucracies, including the government, which may apply to family organizations. This phenomenon has been identified by various researchers as whistleblowing or ethical resistance. It has been identified as the practice of "exposing policies that endanger or defraud the public" (Glazer & Glazer, 1989, p. 11). Walters (1975) identifies the whistle blower as a person within the organization who "having decided at some point that the actions of the organization are immoral, illegal, or inefficient . . . acts on the belief by informing legal authorities or others outside the organization" (p. 26). Specifically, an employee will, "without regard to self, publicly disclose unethical or illegal practices" (Glazer & Glazer, 1989, p. 4). Many cases of whistleblowing have received widespread publicity in recent years. They include, among many others, the exposure of the causes of the Challenger disaster by Morton Thiokol engineers and, earlier, the disclosure of corruption in the New York City Police Department by Frank Serpico. The circumstances of these and other cases are examined to discover whether a parallel for whistleblowing exists within the family organization. In this study, the immoral and illegal act within the family that is examined is limited to parental incest. Thus, the purpose of this study is to gather in-depth data on parental incest and to generate theory about the nature of communication patterns relative to disclosure of incest.

THEORETICAL RATIONALE

The theoretical rationale for this study demonstrates how the organizational structure of the family compares with that of large bureaucracies in the United States. Whistleblowing in the family, then, is a parallel process to whistleblowing in organizations. The theoretical support for the study is the consideration of a family as an organization with specific characteristics of an organization (Anderson & Carter, 1984; Carter & McGoldrick, 1980; Miller, 1989; Parsons, 1964) and the systems approach to psychotherapy (Carter & McGoldrick, 1980; Etizoni, 1964).

Summary of Theoretical Rationale

The rationale presented previously considered the structure of the family in terms of the larger organizational structures in society. Viewing family systems as organizations is fundamental to any analysis of similarities beyond the structural level. For example, the large body of organizational literature can offer pertinent insights on family communication. Therefore, this study examines the nature of disclosure patterns as has been done for large bureaucracies. The organization under consideration in this study is the family; the immoral or illegal act has been limited to parental incest. With few exceptions, incest taboos are universal (de Chesnay, 1985); therefore, limiting the full range of immoral or illegal acts possible to one, incest, is appropriate, considering the universal law of the act. Choosing to focus on incest enabled the investigator to more closely reflect on the wrongdoing recorded in the whistleblowing literature. For example, had alcoholism been selected as the focus, the act of drinking alcohol would not always have been illegal or immoral. Focusing on drug abuse would have met the illegal and immoral criteria, but would have presented serious methodological concerns because of the mind-altering effects of the overuse of drugs. For example, the wrongdoer may have been excused because he was not aware of what he was doing. Incest, on the other hand, being both illegal and immoral and having a body of research literature, was a logical choice for investigation. Prior to this study, data were not available to determine whether the communication of incest in families is analogous to whistleblowing or a decidedly different phenomenon.

Assumptions

1. The family is an organization.
2. Disclosure of incest takes place within a cultural context.
3. Incest survivors are able to recollect and describe their experience to an interviewer.

4. Therapists are accurate reporters of the disclosure reported to them by incest survivors.

5. The data reported by the survivors represent their perspective, regardless of the degree of truthfulness or accuracy of the data. No attempt is made to verify the truthfulness or accuracy of the events reported by the survivors.

Definition of Terms

Whistleblowing: Whistleblowing refers to the act by a person within an organization who, having decided at some point that the actions of the organization are immoral, unethical, illegal, or harmful, informs authorities or others outside the organization.

Incest: Incest refers to sexual relations between culturally defined family members. For the purpose of this study, incest is delimited to any sexual behavior that occurs between parent and child.

Incest survivor: In this study, an incest survivor refers to a female adult who reports having had a sexual relationship with her father during her childhood. For the purpose of this study, the many other categories of incest survivors are not investigated.

Disclosure: For the purpose of this study, disclosure is restricted to mean the first time an incest survivor tells another person, who is not the offender, her incest secret.

Family: For the purpose of this study, family is delimited to an organization of blood relatives.

Etic: Etic is a type of research approach that depends on constructs from the researcher's own perspective. The phenomenon is understood in terms of an external set of standards applied by the researcher.

Emic: Emic is a type of research approach that emphasizes the subjectivity of someone else's life in its own cultural context.

REVIEW OF THE LITERATURE

This chapter is derived from a dissertation that is too lengthy to reprint here. Therefore, the literature review, although comprehensive for whistleblowing, family violence, and incest, is not included in full. However, the key points of the literature link the concepts together and the results section addresses the lineages.

Whistleblowing

The literature on whistleblowing demonstrates that several interrelated social and environmental factors have come into play since the 1960s that have contributed to the emergence of whistleblowing as an identifiable phenomenon. These factors include the struggle over new government regulations of the private sector in the 1960s and 1970s, disillusionment with government and industry's ability to control technological hazards, and the increasing public cynicism about the integrity of federal officials that grew out of the Vietnam conflict and the Watergate scandal (Glazer & Glazer, 1989, p. 11). Along with these factors came a strong belief among some that something could, in fact, be done to rectify illegal or unethical situations. Those who held this belief were the potential whistleblowers. Often described as conservatives operating from high ethical principles, typically, whistleblowers feel that they are justified in exposing unethical organizational or government practices. Self-descriptions by whistleblowers often include a mention of being loyal to their organization, caring deeply about the work of their organizations, and wanting to do the right thing (Glazer & Glazer, 1989, p. 96). They are people with strong belief systems—religious or otherwise—that enable them to withstand the bureaucratic pressures to conform. Usually, whistleblowers try every other means at their disposal to correct the situation before resorting to public disclosure of the problem.

Stewart (1980) identifies the events that occur in a whistleblowing incident and speaks of the progression from awareness of a product or policy believed to be wrong, to action at several levels—from the supervisor to regulatory bodies to the general public via the press. The cost is potentially high, and some whistleblowers might be forced to resign or be fired. The communication events inherent in a whistleblowing incident and the long-term effects of such a disclosure have been studied in nonfamily organizations. Immoral, unethical, and illegal acts do occur in families; however, the family violence literature, and specifically the literature dealing with incest, does not report studies of disclosure.

Family Violence

Detrimental interactions within families are of many types; they differ in form, impact, and presumed cause, as well as in treatment and policy. Both professionals and the media, of late, have compressed these varied events into the generic term *abuse*, which has evolved into a policy concept standing for things done to family members that are regarded by the larger society to be harmful, and regarding which people want to take some kind of remedial or ameliorative action (Gelles & Pedrick, 1985).

As difficult as it has been to document the prevalence/incidence of abuse, intrafamilial abuse is far easier to count than to explain. Studies cluster around documenting the occurrence of abuse and exploring how well victims cope after the abuse, but there is no clear picture of what leads up to the disclosure of the abuse. Intrafamilial abuse research developed in discrete areas and followed distinct eras: physical abuse of children, wife abuse, ritualistic child sexual abuse, and elderly abuse. Initially, the research focused on physical abuse of children. This was, in part, a response to society's increased child welfare concerns in the late 1960s and early 1970s. The women's movement of the mid-1970s supported the next area of research: wife abuse. Finkelhor's (1984) classic work on child sexual abuse represented views that predominated during the late 1970s.

West-Sands (1990) conducted a life history study of the lived experience of incestuous abuse and subsequent exploitation by a therapist. This contributed a richer understanding of the incest experience by identifying the major themes, which were correlated with the four developmental levels of childhood, adolescence, young adulthood, and adulthood. However, no studies had been conducted on the communication events relative to the disclosure of incest.

Summary of the Literature

The major works in this recently emergent field of intrafamilial abuse have contributed to our understanding and appreciation of the occurrence and subsequent coping behaviors of victims. Support systems for victims need services, but we do not have a theoretical perspective as to why people go public, and of equal importance, why some people do not disclose.

Areas of Agreement

Scholars are confident about the theory of whistleblowing in large organizations. However, less is known about whistleblowing in smaller organizations such as the family. This study fills this gap in that the nature of incest as an exploitative and, therefore, immoral and illegal act, makes it an excellent example of a context in which to study whistleblowing. Incest by nature is a family problem and (arguably) the most immoral, illegal family act that tends to be disclosed.

The incest literature does not show how survivors disclose. It is a fact that they do it, but no systematic study of the process of disclosure exists. There is agreement that incest is an exploitative act; building on this agreement of exploitation, investigation of how immoral or unethical practices are disclosed as described in the whistleblowing research has the potential to contribute to the incest literature while also expanding the whistleblowing theory. That is, understanding whistleblowing in incestuous families is a logical next step to understanding whistleblowing in small organizations.

Areas of Disagreement

There are some basic points of disagreement in the whistleblowing literature. The very definition of the term ranges from it being viewed as an accurate description of an antimanagement act to it being considered a flippant term. Although the debate on the most descriptive term for it continues, there is consensus that "it" does, in fact exist. Another area of inconsistency is how the whistleblower himself or herself is viewed. The media often view the whistleblower as a hero; the organization often has a decidedly different view. The more recent works are continuing to expand what is known by contributing additional understandings. The most recent studies have focused on the long-term sequelae of disclosure, for example, ill health including post-traumatic stress disorder (PTSD).

Deficiencies in the Existing Research

There are no theoretically based studies on disclosure of incest that are either random controlled studies or qualitative studies. That is why a naturalistic paradigm for this study was indicated; theories need to be generated. This is not to suggest that there is no theory relative to families, incest, or communication. At this point in time, there is no specific theory on *disclosure of incest* to be tested. This study, utilizing an emic approach, fills the gap. The insider—the survivor—tells from her point of view the steps she followed in disclosure. This will generate the theory that is missing in the literature.

RESEARCH QUESTIONS

The study is designed to answer each of the following research questions:

1. What sequence of events of disclosure is reported by incest survivors who disclose in childhood and incest survivors who disclose in adulthood?
   Subquestion #1: What are the antecedents to disclosure?
   Subquestion #2: What is the content of disclosure?
   Subquestion #3: What is the context of disclosure?
   Subquestion #4: What are the sequelae to disclosure?

2. What is the pattern of disclosure most typically reported to therapists by survivors?
   Subquestion #1: Does this pattern conform to or differ from what has been identified as whistleblowing in large organizations?
   Subquestion #2: How does the disclosure pattern reported by therapists correlate with the disclosure pattern reported in the life histories?

As discussed in the next section, the study is designed so that research question #1 is answered by the life history data, and research question #2 is answered by the survey data.

METHODOLOGY

Sample

Inclusion criteria for the study were (a) female subject, at least 21 years old; (b) someone who disclosed at least 1 year previously, which would provide enough time to articulate the sequelae to disclosure, yet recently enough to recall the events and long enough to have dealt with the distress of disclosure; (c) someone who spoke English well enough for communication with the investigator; and (d) someone who was currently in, or had completed, psychotherapy, as it is not the purpose of this study to work through the emotional issues and distress of incest.

Exclusion criteria for the study were (a) involvement in any organic or drug-induced process that would inhibit recall, (b) severe emotional distress at the time of the interviews, (c) active involvement in legal prosecution of the offender at the time of data collection, and (d) formerly in therapy with the investigator. As the investigator *was* the data collection instrument, the last criterion was needed to minimize confounding variables in the investigator–informant relationship. It is questionable whether refusal or real voluntary participation can be obtained from a client who is or was engaged in a therapeutic relationship with the investigator.

Prior to the collection of the life history data, focus group interviews were held with incest survivors to get a sense of what survivors talk about when they talk about disclosure. Two focus group interviews were conducted, one with a group of seven women and the other with a group of eleven women. These women were members of ongoing support groups for incest survivors. The interviews were not part of a regularly scheduled group session, but a specifically conducted group interview to which members of several ongoing groups, which were run by the same facilitator, were invited. The interviews were each 2 hours in length. Detailed notes were taken by the investigator throughout the interviews. In addition, the regular group facilitator, who was present in the room at the time of the interview, took handwritten notes. Both the investigator and the group facilitator listened for recurring themes, phrases, and terminology used by the survivors. After the interview, notes were compared; the data consisted of themes, possible areas for exploration, and phrases used in describing the incest experiences. The focus group interview data, augmented with clinical practice experience, provided a basis for the construction of the semi-structured interview guide (see Appendix at the end of this chapter) used in the conduct of actual life histories. A pilot study of the interview guide was administered to a survivor who met the study criteria but was not one of the key informants. This pilot indicated that the interview guide was effective in facilitating discussion pertinent to the life history theme of this study—disclosure of incest.

The life histories, which are detailed accounts of a person's life recounted vis-à-vis a particular theme, were then initiated. Because the thematic framework for this investigation is disclosure of incest, two survivors were chosen to be key informants in this study based on their ability to provide an account of the lived experience of incest and subsequent disclosure. The term *key informant* accurately emphasizes the importance of the two survivors in this study. The key informants agreed to spend extensive time with the interviewer, initially recollecting their experience, and then, in subsequent interviews, reviewing interview transcriptions as an accuracy check. Their commitment to this study was extensive in both time and energy. Care was taken to select one key informant who had disclosed during childhood and one who had disclosed as an adult.

Life history interview data were analyzed, categorized, and subjected to both accuracy checks and inter-rater reliability tests. Data from interviews also included a variety of personal documents reviewed during the interviews. This resulted in the final identification of themes and subthemes that emerged from the life histories.

Life History Design

The methodology for a life history is a series of semi-structured interviews by a skilled interviewer who can elicit memories, some of which may be painful. A life history is a detailed account of the development of a person's life for the purpose of identifying a set of common patterns experienced by their peers (Dobbert, 1982; Field & Morse, 1985). The life history method utilizes extensive interviewing and other techniques of inquiry, such as document review, to elicit the emic point of view (from the subject's viewpoint) as the individual is trying to make sense of his or her world (Watson & Watson-Franke, 1985). The insider is essential to understanding the lived experience of the incest survivor. The survivor's reconstruction of the antecedents, content, context, and sequelae of disclosing incest is used for filling theoretical gaps and generating new clinical inventions. The life history provides the cultural context in which the reconstruction takes place. The life history design is unique in its compelling subjectivity and yields insight into a person's life experiences in a culturally defined, experiential context (West-Sands, 1990).

The life history approach for Part 1 of this study is drawn from ethnography. Life histories are often collected by fieldworkers gathering ethnographic data when the key informants' lives particularly reflect the cultural phenomena of interest. The life history is a "retrospective account by the individual of his or her life in whole or part, in written or oral form, that has been elicited or prompted by another person" (Watson & Watson-Franke, 1985, p. 2).

The reason why the life history approach is appropriate for this study, as opposed to other qualitative or quantitative methods, is that the rich detail of the disclosure is outside of the context of the person's life and culture. Utilizing the life history method provides a frame of reference to interpret differences. Of equal importance in choosing the life history method is the fact that this method effectively addresses the ethical concerns inherent in this study. As topics emerged in the interview, there was sufficient time to address not only the content but also the informant's reaction. If, for example, a self-administered questionnaire had been used instead, the informant would not have had the opportunity to talk through sensitive issues. This might have left the informant in a vulnerable position. Further, the answers to questionnaire items would not necessarily provide the opportunity to understand the context of the situation, thus doing an injustice to the informant's perspective.

Life History as an Emic Approach

The life history has been used for more than 65 years in social scientific research, as a source of information about the human condition (Watson & Watson-Franke, 1985). Fundamentally, the life history is one distinctive type of personal document. As a generic category, personal documents are any expressive production of individuals that can clarify their view of self or of their situation as they see it. Personal document review has long been recognized as an effective means of accessing the individual's perspective at the time. To understand why a person does something or does not do something, it is necessary to understand how the situation looked to that person. A summary look at the historical and theoretical development of life history as a research methodology will lay the foundation for its being the method of choice in this study.

As early as 1913, anthropologists were using the life history as a major source of information about a culture. In discussing his research of 1913, Radin (1920) stated that his aim was to obtain an "inside view" of another culture, told in the words of an insider, to avoid destruction of the subjective value inherent in the events described (p. 383). A landmark study in 1920 (Thomas & Znaniecki, 1920–1927) is credited as being the publication that spurred interest in personal documents for the purpose of research. After 1920, studies using personal documents proliferated in both anthropology and sociology. The life history was regarded as "the perfect type of sociological material" (Thomas & Znaniecki, 1920–1927, pp. 1832–1833) to characterize the life of a social group. The 1930s saw the emergence of a field study within anthropology that would come to have a significant positive impact on the status of life history in research (Watson & Watson-Franke, 1985, pp. 6–7); the culture and personality school of thought resulted from the merger of psychology and anthropology. One of its prominent advocates, Edward Sapir (1934), believed that the merger made sense on many levels. Studying culture as a grand, impersonal whole was detrimental to the explanation of how an individual behaves and how individuals behave toward each other. Sapir (1934) saw the merger as fitting, because the more one attempts to understand culture, "the more it seems to take on the characteristics of a personality organization" (p. 412).

Refinement of the life history method continued into the 1940s. In his *Criteria for the Life History*, Dollard (1935) put forth a combination of principles from cultural research and psychoanalysis. This blending was designed to decrease confusion in the use of the life history. As a Freudian analyst, Dollard brought much preoccupation with the imposition of theoretical constructs to the interpretive process; however, despite the analytical skill demanded by Dollard for the life history, he is acknowledged as genuinely improving the fieldwork methodology (Langness & Frank, 1981, pp. 20–21).

Utilizing the sophistication that Dollard (1935) brought to the life history, many researchers (Kardiner, 1945; Simmons, 1942) contributed information from the insider's life experience. Simmons's work is illustrative of the time:

> In Sun Chief, Simmons (1942) did employ the concept of personality in relation to culture in his analysis of the life history of Don Talayesva, a Hopi Indian. The idea of "adjustments" an individual makes to the limitations imposed by his biological capabilities, physical environment, society, and culture plays a crucial role in Simmons' analytical scheme. Realizing that an analysis of an entire personality with his formula might prove superficial, he attempted an in-depth "situational analysis" using the concept of adjustment . . . recognized as a major contribution to the growing interest in the life history, both for its thoughtful analysis and because Simmons provided the immediate context of the document, including a description of the relationship between the narrator and the ethnographer. (Kluckhohn, 1943; Watson & Watson-Franke, 1985, p. 8)

From the 1950s on, the life history was used in many research areas, including individual adjustment to culture conflict (Spradley, 1969), role analysis (Hughes, 1965, 1974), identity conflict and self-appraisal (Watson, 1970), and individual adaptation within a sociocultural system (Aberle, 1967).

Given its ability to provide a comprehensive, holistic examination of the subjective life experience, the life history method is the most appropriate design for this study. This method was used for the purpose of identifying a set of recurring patterns experienced by the survivor, which may also have been experienced by her peers (Dobbert, 1982; Field & Morse, 1985). Life history investigations captured lived experiences as seen from the point of view of the individual. Because the life history document is one of subjectivity or perspective, through which an individual articulates her world and reflects her personal view of her life as she understands it (West-Sands, 1990), the life history is a method that is well suited to seeking the explanation of life in a family organization from an insider's perspective.

The Researcher as Instrument

In naturalistic designs, such as a life history, the primary instrument is the researcher, because it is only through the skill of the interviewer that accurate data are collected. Classical anthropology and sociology field research has rarely used any instrument other than the researcher (Lincoln & Guba, 1985). When conducting research from the naturalistic paradigm, it is virtually impossible to construct a priori an instrument that is sufficiently adaptable and comprehensive to address the all-encompassing realities that will be encountered (Lincoln & Guba, 1985).

Humans are uniquely qualified to serve as instruments in naturalistic inquiries for several reasons. Only humans can sense and respond to interpersonal and environmental cues; this responsiveness to the situation allows explication of the situation to the reader. Admittedly imperfect, humans are nonetheless adaptable to multiple variables, which a written questionnaire is not. A human instrument is capable of grasping phenomena within its context and of revealing the holistic perspective.

Watson and Watson-Franke (1985) note that there are key issues associated with using the investigator as an instrument. These issues should be dealt with in the write-up of the final report and should address the following questions: What is the relationship that occurred? What are the circumstances in which the informant related the life history? What information is volunteered and what is given in response to direct questioning? How does the investigator motivate the informant to relate her life history? What are the investigator's preconceptions and theoretical commitments that might influence collection, analysis, and interpretation of data? In addition to these issues, Langness and Frank (1981) assert that personality traits of the investigator influence the content and process of the life history. Life history investigators must engage in self-examination to gain insight into their own personality, beliefs, and values if they are to determine how much of their work reflects themselves and how much is the informant's view of reality. These questions are discussed in Chapter 4 of this volume.

Along with this notion of personality influences, this study illustrates the need to consider occupational and role performance influences. The investigator for this study is academically trained as a psychotherapist, holding a Master of Science degree in advanced clinical psychiatric nursing, with family systems analysis as the area of concentration. American Nurse Association (ANA) board-certified as a clinical specialist in psychiatric–mental health nursing, she has maintained a private practice in psychotherapy for 19 years. Adult survivors of childhood sexual abuse including, but not limited to, incest have been seen in both long-term psychotherapy and crisis intervention. In addition, the investigator facilitates group counseling sessions for survivors and conducts training workshops for professionals. The researcher has had extensive experience in teaching courses on psychotherapeutic interviewing techniques at both the undergraduate and graduate level. Clinical experience and specialized training in working with adult survivors of childhood sexual abuse augment the investigator's basic interviewing skills.

For studies in which the researcher serves as the primary instrument, issues of validity, reliability, and pilot testing are interrelated. Naturalistic methods do not require pilot tests in the same way as do quantitative studies. Pilot tests are necessary in quantitative studies to establish the validity and reliability of the instrument, among other things. In qualitative studies such as the life history, however, the validity and reliability considerations are met within the context of the interviewer's skills (Lincoln & Guba, 1985; Watson & Watson-Franke, 1985). The investigator has experience interviewing people in a variety of settings: her office, their homes, hospitals, and public locations in crisis situations. The investigator has treated approximately 20 incest survivors. These survivors have discussed the fact that they have disclosed as well as some of the events associated with disclosure. Therefore, the investigator has a clinical basis for framing the subproblems for the study in the areas of antecedent, content, context, and sequelae. The investigator also has extensive experience audiotaping psychotherapy sessions, transcribing tapes, and interpreting themes in context. Thus, the researcher is well qualified to serve as the instrument for this study.

Interview Guide

To examine the feasibility of the semi-structured interview guide as shown in the Appendix at the end of this chapter, the investigator conducted a preliminary test with a survivor who was not part of the study but who met the eligibility criteria. The interviewee was able to answer, elaborate, and deviate within the limits of the questions posed. This preliminary testing of the interview guide demonstrated two major points: (a) The guide was effective in facilitating discussion of life history within the thematic framework, that of disclosure of incest, and (b) the time required would be more than initially anticipated by the investigator. However, the quality of the responses war-ranted the time invested. No questions were eliminated, and no questions were added as a result of the interview.

Conduct of Interviews

The selection of key informants, determination of setting, length of inter-views, and the interview format were all consistent with the life history method. Using key informants means using the best informants, that is, those individuals best able to talk about the phenomenon within their life context. Key Informant #1, who heard about the study at a lecture given by the investigator during the planning stage of the study, asked to participate. As she very clearly met the study criteria, she was accepted. The selection of Key Informant #2 took place after two interviews were completed with Key Informant #1. This allowed for purposeful sampling. For example, the age, economic status, educational status, religion, and ethnicity of the indi-vidual chosen to be Key Informant #2 would be different from those of Key Informant #1. In addition, the time of disclosure would differ: Key Infor-mant #1 disclosed during childhood; Key Informant #2 disclosed in adult-hood. The investigator contacted a colleague who counsels incest survivors. She explained the study, including the provisions for protection of human subjects, and requested referral of a survivor who met the criteria. The refer-ring therapist explained the study to Key Informant #2, who was interested in participating. The investigator made telephone contact with the woman and scheduled an appointment. As far as possible, as is consistent with the naturalistic paradigm, sampling for diversity guided these informant selec-tion decisions. However, both informants had to meet the overall criteria the investigator had established for this study.

Human Subjects Approval

The use of human subjects for the study was approved by the Rutgers University institutional review board (IRB) before data collection began. A potential benefit to the key informant participating in this study was that talking through often helps people make more sense of a traumatic experi-ence and fosters the healing process that the survivor has already begun with her therapist. Although it is sometimes difficult for people to talk about pain-ful memories, it is more common for people to benefit from the experience of talking it out with a knowledgeable and compassionate listener. Catharsis as an outcome of naturalistic inquiry has been recognized by ethicists and researchers (de Chesnay, 1991).

A potential risk to the key informant involved remembering things that might have been uncomfortable. Supportive strategies were employed throughout the study. For example, if at any point during the interview the informant's stress level increased, the interviewer, based on her professional assessment of the situation, stopped the interview, gave anxiety reduction directives to the informant, or redirected the conversation. If at any point during the study, the informant wished to withdraw, her wishes would be respected without consequence to her. However, neither of the key informants withdrew.

Setting

The actual data collection took place in various locations in New Jersey mutually agreed on by the key informant and the interviewer. All interviews were audiotaped for later transcription. Most interviews with Key Informant #1 were held in a private office on a college campus. One interview was conducted in a park, and three briefer interviews were over the telephone, as the informant had relocated during the study. The college setting was suggested by the informant; the significance of the choice became apparent to the investigator later. Interviews with Key Informant #2 were held at an inner city YWCA in private offices. This location was chosen by the informant and was, the investigator learned later, a very special place for her.

The purposive sampling not only resulted in diversity among the informants with regard to economic status, education, occupation, and ethnicity but also reflected the choice of settings for the interviews. The setting itself became part of the data collected. For example, Key Informant #1 spoke of her parents communicating to her throughout her childhood that she was not an able student; no discussions about college/career plans took place as had been the case with her older brothers. The interviews for this study took place on the college campus where, as an adult, Key Informant #1 completed her education, graduating with honors.

Key Informant #2 chose the YWCA for all interviews; it was the very building where she first disclosed the incest.

The semi-structured interview guide was used during the actual conduct of the life history interviews. The questions served as a general framework for eliciting data about the key informants' lives, cultural background, and the events surrounding the disclosure of the incest. The initial questions were general in nature and, in part, served to put the informants at ease.

As the interviews progressed and rapport was established, the questions became more focused on the sequences of communication in disclosure. Maximum flexibility was permitted, allowing the key informants to set the pace and depth of the interview. Cultural data, for example, ethnicity, educational level, and rules, were specifically elicited in several of the questions.

To interpret data within the cultural context, the investigator maximized the chance of differences rather than controlled for differences. This was accomplished in part by purposive sampling. The emic approach supported the eliciting of key informants' perspectives as insiders. Throughout the data collection process, the investigator examined her own theoretical and cultural biases, personal beliefs and values, personality, and communication strategies to assess the reliability and validity of the instrument. After the collection of data, during the analysis, the questions identified by Watson and Watson-Franke (1985) were discussed with colleagues and committee members, and efforts were made to separate emic and etic views. In addition, informants reviewed the data during the analysis phase as an additional accuracy check.

An important component for novice researchers is supervision or consultation with an experienced researcher. The importance of ongoing supervision is illustrated by the following occurrence in this study. Early in the conduct of the first life history with Key Informant #1, during an inter-rater reliability check, it was pointed out to the investigator that she was engaged in what appeared to be a psychotherapy session with the informant. The data recorded verbatim were carefully reviewed with a methodologist, who is also a psychotherapist, and corrective strategies were planned. For example, the past as well as the substance of the questions needed to be brought into a sharper focus. The focus would enable a greater depth of understanding but would need to be continually balanced with just enough latitude to accommodate other pertinent information. That the strategy was effectively implemented was evidenced by the clearer historical data gathered in the next interview. The conduct of the interview also permitted the informant to share the following pertinent data: Since interview #1, she had written a confrontational letter to her abusive parents. It is a constant challenge for the investigator to gain such insights and admit the influence of personal variables to the reader, so that the life history may be evaluated in the light of known biases (Langness & Frank, 1981).

Although the primary means of data collection was interviewing, it should be noted that in the context of the life history, it is helpful to check with any other sources that can verify facts. For example, when Key Informant #1 stated that her parents continued to write her "hate letters . . . and I keep every one of them," a review of the documents (in this case, the letters) was deemed appropriate to the method and was performed. Examples of other documents reviewed in this study include diary entries made by Key Informant #2 during her high school years and some writings done the day after she was raped. This triangulation serves the purpose of verifying interview data with other sources.

The interviews with both key informants varied in length from 1½ to 3 hours. At the end of each interview, the investigator summarized the interview. Summarization invited the informant to react to the material; remarking on the validity of the investigator's constructions provided a member check for validity of the information obtained. Summation also induced the informant to elaborate on certain points (Lincoln & Guba, 1985). Throughout the data collection phase, efforts were made to assess data reliability and validity. For example, the investigator asked for the same information at repeated intervals. This enabled the investigator to assess the reliability of the data given (Langness & Frank, 1981). An illustration of this technique is inquiring about a topic already discussed as if seeking clarification. Such an inquiry might be conducted as follows: "I realize we've covered this before, but I'm not sure I'm clear. Can you tell me about it again?"

The data provided were then compared with those given previously to assess reliability. Immediately following the interview, or as soon as possible, the investigator wrote reflective notes in a log and arranged for the interview tapes to be transcribed (specifics regarding selection of transcriptionists are discussed later in the chapter). The investigator then analyzed the data for the predominant themes. Analysis of the tapes aided in deciding how to proceed with the remaining interviews. For example, when the informant's recollection was vague, clarifying questions were needed to address inconsistencies noted in the previous interview. The remaining interviews were conducted, and the tapes were transcribed and analyzed. When all the interviews were completed, the cultural data were organized chronologically for each key informant. The typology, which is a conceptual map of the themes and categories that emerge from the data, was then developed. Next, it was determined whether each of the categories was saturated—meaning that certain themes predominated. At this point, the investigator conducted accuracy assessments by checking the data with each key informant. In addition, an inter-rater reliability assessment was performed. Three therapists, who are colleagues of the investigator, independently reviewed the data. The total time spent in data review with experts for the purpose of inter-rater reliability was in excess of 25 hours. Based on the categories that emerged from the data, the final literature review was then completed.

Transcriptionists

Because of the nature of the study and the sensitivity of the data, only professional medical transcriptionists were used to transcribe the audiotapes. This
was very clearly stated in the IRB application. The investigator felt strongly
about this being the only ethical way to handle the data. The investigator,
a psychotherapist, had experience of having steps transcribed in the past,
although she had been transcribing on her own for the past several years.
Medical transcriptionists were contacted and interviewed over the telephone. The study was described, and confidentiality, time table, and fees
were reviewed. The transcriptionist selected had recently been featured in a
women's newspaper, in a special edition of women entrepreneurs. She had
a well-established company and was known by the medical records departments of local hospitals. Several days after she had been given the tapes, she
called the investigator with concerns about the confidentiality of the data.
She wanted assurance that the informant had been advised that a transcriptionist would be hearing the tapes. Although this information had been given
to her during the first telephone contact, she absolutely refused to listen to
the tapes. An unsigned copy of the informed consent was given to her—the
signed copy had the full name of the informant, so it could not be shown to
the transcriptionist—as well as the IRB approval form. After several more
days had passed, the investigator contacted her over the telephone. She
reported having some mechanical difficulties and said she would call "next
week." The investigator called again, attempting to arrange for the delivery
of the transcriptions; the transcriptionist was hostile, stating that she had
personal health problems and could not deliver the tapes, nor was the cou-
rier service available. The investigator offered to pick up the work, to which
the transcriptionist replied, "that's just not possible . . . I can't travel back to
the office." Two days later, she personally delivered the transcriptions. She
appeared tense and on guard. She refused to sit, and she and the investigator stood in the investigator's office. During the conversation, which lasted
about 15 minutes, the transcriptionist disclosed that she had had "some
problems" years ago. She did not wish to elaborate; however, with guidance
from the investigator, who was prepared to offer referrals as appropriate, she
did share that she was currently "seeing someone" about the matter.

When reviewing the transcriptions later, listening to the tape while reading, the investigator noted that profanity was omitted from the transcription.
For example, "Fuck you! You goddamn bastard! Get the hell out of here!"
became: "Get the h__ out of here." The transcriptionist later called to say that
she was "too busy with several large accounts" to do more tapes. That same

week, a large business advertisement for her company appeared in the local newspaper. In a study (Alexander et al., 1989) involving document review at a rape crisis center, it was noted that the research assistants required specific debriefing time and support measures after reading the incident reports. The transcriptionist was replaced for this study. Support measures and debriefing were initiated with the new transcriptionist. In addition, the investigator personally did some of the transcribing.

Data Analysis

A series of analytic strategies was utilized to systematically extrapolate meaning from the data. Analytic techniques, which begin concretely and progress to conceptual, included unitizing, noting patterns, categorizing, noting relations, and building conceptual coherence (Lincoln & Guba, 1985; Miles & Huberman, 1984). Units of information were identified; a unit is the smallest piece of information that can stand alone. It has meaning in the absence of additional information (West-Sands, 1990). The units were written on index cards and coded with the interview number, which yielded the data and the source, for example, informant, personal correspondence, family album, and so forth.

After identifying units of data, the next step was pattern noting. The data were continually reviewed to note the emergence of frequently repeated themes, explanations, constructs, or relationships. Themes that emerged were identified and word labels selected that represented the category of information; categories were collections of cards that related to the same content or property (Lincoln & Guba, 1985). Rules were devised to justify inclusion of data unit cards into a category and to ensure the internal consistency of the set.

The first step in categorization was to select the top card from a complete set of data unit reads; the card was read and its contents noted, and it was set aside. The second card was read, its content evaluated as to whether it was similar in content or emotion to the first card. If it was similar, it was added to the first card stack, and if not, a new category was started. Each successive card was assessed, comparing and contrasting the data unit with prior categories and adding new categories as needed (Lincoln & Guba, 1985).

Categories were reviewed repeatedly, with the investigator remaining open to discriminating evidence (Ammon-Gaberson & Piantanida, 1988). The goal of this procedure, the noting relations phase of data analysis, was the acquisition of homogeneous categories. The investigator tried to recognize dissimilarities within the categories and consider the plausibility of a separate theme's existence. Repeated reviews of the categories aided in the recognition of data that did not fit the pattern. These misfits were then removed and entered into an existing category, or they became a new category. This process continued until all the data fit homogenously into categories (Lincoln & Guba, 1985; Miles & Huberman, 1984).

To establish conceptual coherence, categories were again examined, but this time keeping in mind the question, What commonalities do the units of the category share? The commonalities were at a more abstract level than the initially chosen label. A construct label that depicted the content and emotion of the category was assigned; it captured the theme or essence of the category. The constructs identified contributed to factor isolation for the development of factor-isolating theory building in subsequent studies.

Finally, as an accuracy check, the construct labels were reviewed by the key informants to ascertain accurate representation. Traditional reductionist measures of reliability and validity are not appropriate in naturalistic paradigm research. There are, however, correlates; the accuracy discussed earlier most closely resembles validity. Validity of data depends on prolonged engagement or time of sufficient duration and intensity to gain understanding (Lincoln & Guba, 1985). The investigator must be accepted into the informant's culture and internal world to obtain accurate, credible data, and this acceptance process takes time. The skills, interpersonal and otherwise, of the investigator facilitate this process.[1]

RESULTS

The results of this study are presented in the dissertation in two parts. In the first part, life histories presented in this chapter and data from both key informants are presented with identification of the themes that emerged. The literature relevant to each theme is presented. As is consistent with the study design, the life history data are presented in a narrative style. Additional data, in the form of representative quotations of the key informants, are provided in the appendix of the dissertation and are not repeated here.

Summary of Themes

From the interviews with the key informants, four themes and eight sub-themes emerged that represent the dynamics of the lived experience of incest and its subsequent disclosure. It is important to note that these themes were concurrent, sequential, and/or interrelated; the artificial separation of themes for discussion herein is for clarity in presentation of results. The overall thematic framework for this study is disclosure of incest. Therefore, each of the 12 themes that emerged contributes to the composite picture of the cultural context in which the incest and disclosure took place. As is typical for the reporting of life history data, a narrative format is followed as much as possible. Following the life histories, each theme is discussed and brief quotations, which were selected from the data set, are given as examples. Following the quotations are elaborated descriptions that clarify the context of the preceding quotation. The life history data reported here were derived by relying solely on the key informants and their own personal documents. Although they are not presented as historical facts, life data are the best source of the survivor's perspective. The following poem, written by Key Informant #2 at the age of 15 years, serves to answer the question, Are these stories true? In the words of the informant, "It is what I believe."

I have something I want to say. I don't know why I want to say it or even how to say it. I've begun to think a lot about it lately. I've realized I don't know for sure what I want to say. But if it's so important, why can't I say it? Because it is so important to me? It's what I believe. If this is so, why should I believe and you won't understand. Or do I just think you won't understand? You want to understand. But how can you understand if I don't and I believe it. There are no words to tell you how I feel.

THE STORIES

Key Informant #1: Allyson

The informant is hereafter referred to by the pseudonym she selected for use in this study. Allyson Kenny is a 29-year-old White woman. Her father is Jewish, and her mother a Roman Catholic, although neither is practicing. Her father, an engineer, describes his ethnicity as American; her mother, a freelance illustrator, is Russian and Hungarian. Allyson has been married for 4 years and has one child, a son, who is 2 years old. During the course of this study, she discovered that she was pregnant. Allyson is a strikingly attractive woman who could easily be mistaken for a teenager because of her young appearance. However, in her business attire, which is very fashionable and complete with tasteful jewelry and artistically applied makeup, she appears to be in her early twenties. Five feet two inches tall and 110 pounds, she has slightly longer than shoulder-length hair that is naturally dark blond; it is permed in the popular long curled strands. Allyson is a college graduate employed in a significant managerial position in a large health care support industry. Her husband has been a homemaker since the birth of their first child.

Allyson is the third of five children; she has two older brothers and a younger brother and sister. Her father, a consulting engineer, was transferred to Europe when Allyson was 5 years old. The family accompanied him and lived in Europe for 2 years. The first 7 years of Allyson's life are not particularly memorable, being neither positive nor negative, except for a clear memory of her parents being very strict. She recalls being an exceptionally beautiful child; photographs confirm this. The three children were always dressed alike, she in the girl version of her brothers' outfits. The clothing was of very good quality. Both parents fussed over their beautiful daughter.

> I looked like a little fairy, a little pixy doll. I was very small; I was always very small. At that time I was constantly told that I was very lovely, and I can't remember anything bad about my relationship with either of my parents.

Allyson's younger brother, who is 6 years younger than her, was born in Europe. When the family returned to the United States, they settled in a fine home in an upper middle-class suburban neighborhood. Almost immediately, Allyson's mother began working outside of the home on a part-time basis. Allyson remembers that the incest began at age eight or nine; she also very much remembers not feeling beautiful any more.

> It seems like around the time I started going through that awkward stage, about nine. You know you're not so cute anymore, you're starting to get lanky, a little awkward-looking and stuff. It seemed to happen whenever I was no longer so beautiful, I started to have, kind of like, a little bit of crooked nose, and the eyes were sunk, and I wasn't so beautiful. I had very, very crooked teeth. And all of a sudden I started to change, and I think that's when it all started it—father abusing me, and my eldest brother abusing me—all started around the same time . . . . I was eight or nine.

The sexual abuse by her father continued for more than 10 years. Allyson particularly remembers Saturdays. Her friends called her Cinderella because she had a long list of chores to do while caring for her younger siblings. Her older brothers "took out the trash" for their chore and then went out with their friends. The home was large and beautiful, exquisitely furnished, and regularly well cared for. Allyson spent Saturdays scrubbing toilets, washing clothes, cleaning the kitchen, and enduring sexual abuse by her father, who did not work on Saturdays.

On those occasions when both parents were out, her oldest brother, Lloyd, was in charge. Lloyd, 5 years older than Allyson, exercised his authority during these times by subjecting Allyson to numerous abuses.

> He [Lloyd] would tie me to a chair and punish and abuse me. He would not allow me privileges until he was finished sodomizing me.

When Allyson was in the sixth grade, Lloyd, who was in high school, was having many problems.

> He got involved in a lot of drugs, not just grass but mescaline, acid, things like that. He got in trouble breaking into the school, was put on probation, had to do community service. This was a big, dark side of my family.

This was a very significant experience, as it brought the family to the attention of the authorities.

> It was very traumatic . . . . my mother was very dramatic because they made my parents go to family counseling, and they refused, so my brother went, but my parents didn't go. They left a few sessions . . . my mother said the doctor didn't know anything . . . knew nothing about *her* son. They would have no part of it [counseling]. That's a classic theme in my family; when I went for counseling at another point in my life [age 16 for anorexia], they would have no part of it; in fact, the counselor stopped seeing me because my family would not come in, and she felt that she could not go any further with me without my parents' involvement, and they would have no part of it . . . we were supposed to be perfect; she [mother] wanted the Camelot family.

From about the age of 8, Allyson remembers feeling that she "didn't fit in with other girls." She remembers going to join the Brownies, but it didn't last long. Her mother wanted her out of the organization; Allyson was overprotected and not allowed to go anywhere other than school. It was, however, the Brownie leader who asked Allyson's mother to remover her from the troop. "The leader didn't like me . . . I wasn't like the hip chicks.

I was quiet and mousy." Allyson was actually relieved to be removed from the troop; she felt very out of place, different from the other members, and had no sense of belonging to the group. To this day, Allyson struggles with these same feelings. Around the same time as the Brownie experience, Allyson attempted another "out-of-the-family" activity, for which she had her mother's permission.

> My mother considered herself very liberal regarding religion. Lloyd was BarMitzvah, and was the end of it; by the time we all came along, they just said whatever you want to be, you be.

In this out-of-family venture, Allyson attended a Christian Bible class with a neighborhood girl her age.

> I came home talking love, and Jesus loves me, and she [mother] said, "That's the end of that. Honey, you are out of there." She wouldn't let me go back.

Melissa was born when Allyson was 8 years old. Allyson had always wanted a baby sister and was "thrilled" to finally have her. Much of the baby's care was delegated to Allyson, who accepted the caretaker role lovingly. "I absolutely adored her!" For Allyson, Melissa became the beautiful part of her life.

From the age of 8 approximately, until she was literally thrown out of the house at age 23, Allyson was subjected to physical abuse by her mother. Because of the beatings and her mother's obese size and strength, Allyson lived in fear of being hurt.

> She [mother] was always flipping out. She would verbally abuse me while beating the hell out of me . . . One time she was lying right on top of me beating me with her fists. My father was standing in the doorway watching.

Looking at her father standing there making no effort to intervene triggered a realization: There was no payoff for what she endured with her father. He would do nothing to help her. Although all the children were targets of the verbal abuse, according to Allyson, the words used were more vulgar and hurtful when directed at her.

> My mother called me a slut and a whore. She'd say things like, "You can't wait to get it in your mouth." To my sister she might suggest that she [sister] was being "a little loose."

It was the norm in the household for the children to call their parents by their first names, Albert and Edith. "That's just the way it was."

In her first year of high school, at the age of 13, Allyson began running track. Running was to continue to be a major way of coping throughout high school. Her weight dropped to about 80 pounds. She ran before school, at school during lunch time, after school, and weekends. Usual teenage girl behaviors such as borrowing clothes, sleepovers, and parties were forbidden. Although school friends were permitted in the house, the children were not encouraged to bring them.

Actually, they [school friends] didn't want to be in our house. They thought it was strange . . . They were amazed that we called our parents Edith and Albert. I guess it *was* strange when you think about it—to be so controlling and then to be *Edith and Albert*.

Allyson describes herself as being incredibly naïve and sheltered. It was not until she was in high school that she started seeing other families and began putting things together.

I got to be around my best friend's family. A wonderful family and a wonderful mother, a fine woman. She was really like a second mother to me. And *my* mother walked into this girl's sweet sixteen birthday party and dragged me out of the house because I did something bad or just that she was mad at me and humiliated me. This was an existing pattern; the family was very closed; there was not a lot of anything allowed; no going out, no going in . . . I wasn't allowed to date until I was eighteen without a chaperone. My brothers, Lloyd and Steve, chaperoned me for my prom. My brother chaperoned me throughout high school.

A few days before her 16th birthday, Allyson reports that she was "grounded" for walking home alone from a friend's house. Later that night, Edith opened the door to Allyson's bedroom and threw her birthday present, ice skates, on the floor. That was her "sweet sixteen." Six months later, Edith made a beautiful sugar-cube corsage and a cake for a friend's 16th birthday; from Allyson's perspective, Edith knew how to hurt her emotionally as well as physically.

It was during high school that Allyson says her "conscious life" began. At age 14 or 15, she first realized that her father's behavior was not right.

I was in high school and somebody said something, and all of a sudden it kind of clicked. Like, "*Wow*, you know, this is happening. And this isn't cool; this isn't the right thing that should be happening. This is not what happens in families.

After this realization, her life became a "huge race." She was constantly in a hurry and could not sit still. Running was a big part of her life.

I'd do anything to get out of that house. I ran every morning. It was the one thing that was mine; I achieved something with that. It kept me out of the house. Track was great.

Coping became an everyday struggle and remains so even today. Her exercising intensified as did her eating disorder. These years were character-ized by fear and confusion. She tried to make sense of what was happening in her life. The sexual abuse by her father continued; he became even more daring, entering her room and abusing her as Edith worked at her desk in another room. The sexual assaults took place throughout the house: in bed-rooms, bathrooms, wherever and whenever her father wanted. Allyson was very confused by many things happening to and around her. She remembers thinking that it was a little strange that her brother Steve, a teenage boy, would want to crawl into bed with his mother every morning after his shower.

He just stayed on one side of the bed; there was never anything to it, but I did think it was not typical for a teenage boy.

In her senior year of high school, Allyson wrote a term paper that was singled out as outstanding and sent by the faculty to a nationally known university, which was doing research on the topic. No one asked Allyson how it was that she produced such an accomplished paper. She had intimate knowledge of her subject: incest. And no one asked.

Things began to sort of make sense. I thought: That's it, that's my job. My job is to keep this family together, because if I open my mouth it would be like I split the whole family out.

It was not long, however, before the bulimia, and with it, the purg-ing, began. That was a very intense period in Allyson's life. When she real-ized what incest was, and that it was happening to her, she does not recall thinking about how to cope with the situation. She remembers her atten-tion being focused on running, gymnastics, and her friends. These activities gave her something to think about and helped her get out of the house. From the time her "conscious life" began until about age 17, she tried to stay busy. This is also the point at which the multiplicity of her life story recollections can be seen. The order of the events that occurred during these years has blurred for Allyson. This may be, in part, the result of her overall weakened condition from the bulimia. The stress of events also contributes to the blurring. In addition, multiple stories reflect reality and can, in fact, imply the truth. Therefore, no attempt was made by the researcher to specify one version or the chronology. The events related by Allyson in several interviews were grouped by the researcher in the time frame of age 16 through 18 years.

Her eating disorder was intensified. As was the norm in her home, her parents regularly spied on their children, especially Allyson, and that is how they discovered she was bulimic. She was taken to a counselor, whom she saw for 6 months. Allyson discussed the bulimia; she disclosed the incest. She does not remember if she told the counselor that her father was still abusing her, or if she framed it in past tense. It was not difficult to tell the counselor about the incest because she was a stranger, because she was not close to the family. Telling really "wasn't a big deal." The counselor asked the parents to come to therapy with Allyson. The parents refused, and the counselor refused to see Allyson. The first disclosure did not change the situation. Allyson remembers this time as being unclear and confusing. Clarity entered the picture when she realized that she had something very important that needed her attention.

> It became very apparent to me when I hit seventeen and I thought to myself: I have a little sister there what am I going to do about that? This was a very crucial issue to me . . . her well-being. I knew then, I realized then that he was going to have contact with her. And it was imperative, it was in the forefront of my mind, that I had to save her from him [father].

Allyson's intense concern about Melissa's safety began when Melissa was 9 years old, the age at which Allyson's abuse began. Her fears became realities. One day Allyson walked into the bedroom she shared with Melissa and found her father sitting on the bed with his hands up under the covers. Allyson flew into a rage. She went over to her father and spoke to him in a way she had never done before:

> You don't touch her! You stay the fuck away from her . . . I'll keep my mouth shut about what you do to me, but you stay away from her!

Edith was working in the other room at the time of this confrontation. Allyson talked with Melissa, who confirmed that Albert had been "bothering" her. Allyson felt that it was extremely important for Melissa to have correct information about what was happening. She was consumed with protecting her sister.

> She really had to know that it is not right, it is not okay for people to do this to other people, especially with your father. Later on it's okay with men, men you are in love with; all of the things are okay then, but this what he was doing was not right.

Allyson made a deal with Albert to ensure Melissa's safety: "This is how it's going to be. You stay away from her, and I'll keep my mouth shut about what you do to me." She notes that she was confused a great deal during this time. She did not understand why this was happening to her. She did not understand why her mother, who was only 35 feet away from the bedroom, did nothing. Allyson rationalized that Edith must have been abused as a child in her own alcoholic family. Allyson continued to be clear about one thing: It was her job to keep the family together.

Immediately after the incident with Albert and Melissa, Allyson went to see Lloyd who was away at college. She went to enlist Lloyd's help in protecting Melissa. She disclosed the incest to him. Allyson was weak and tired from the bulimia; she turned to Lloyd because she saw him as powerful and strong.

> I didn't know what might have to be done. Maybe we'd need to get some of his big friends together and go in there and get her out . . . I just didn't know.

Although verbally supportive, Lloyd, to the best of Allyson's knowledge, took no action. Allyson felt confident that Albert had heeded her threat, but the sexual abuse continued with Allyson. She became more ill with her eating disorder. Several months later, weakened and tired of trying so hard, she disclosed the incest to her second oldest brother, Steve.

> Sometimes I think about it [disclosing to Steve]. I feel very guilty because I feel that I did it for myself. I didn't do it for the right reasons. I didn't do it because I was helping somebody else. I did it because I wanted him to wake up. It's like: "Wake up, Steve. You know you're not living in Camelot; this is the little shithole you're living in and I want you to see it for what it is. Stop going around thinking it's so glorious. Your father molested me. . . You don't know shit about my life . . . ."

This third disclosure did not seem to affect the situation, from Allyson's perspective, except that Allyson felt guilty about telling Steve the painful information. She thought of the conversation as being futile. One thing that had been changing was the family composition. Lloyd had moved away to college; Steve was involved in the dining table career discussions and would also leave for college. Allyson would never have career discussions with her parents, or with anyone else for that matter. Looking back at this time, Allyson is amazed that she never realized she had to think about her life and her work. She was incredibly involved in keeping the family together and protecting Melissa. No one in the family encouraged Allyson, as had been done for her brothers; the brothers were seriously sat down at the dining-room table where college catalogs were studied. For Allyson, the dining-room table was just a study in more family rigidity.

The elegant dining room was the setting for daily family meals. Although the children would have preferred an earlier schedule, the evening meal was at 8 p.m. It was always formal: All family members came to the table dressed up; no one left the table, which was complete with cloth napkins, before everyone was finished. The scene was reenacted nightly. It was picture perfect. The picture did not show that the oldest daughter was starving herself to near-death at this bountiful table.

After graduating from high school, Allyson entered a 2-year program at the community college near her home. She continued to live with her parents and younger brother and sister. Allyson's relationship with Edith was stormy, and fights between the two were frequent. Allyson was weary from the burden of so many years and from bulimia. She let her guard down.

I had just about had it. My life was extremely hard. I was very involved with my bulimia . . . . I had just had it with keeping secrets and pretending. I was very tired. I was at a drive-in movie with my best friend, the one whose mother was so good to me, and I just told her what my father had done. She almost died. She was astonished because she thought we were the perfect family. She knew my mother was hard on me, but she had no idea.

It was a very hard final year at school. In a psychology class, the students were discussing sexual abuse. Allyson remembers them joking and being very insensitive. She finally shouted out, "Look this is not funny! This happened to me and this is not funny." She ran from the room feeling very much alone. This disclosure was memorable for Allyson because it reinforced her belief that no one understands the pain.

Just before her last semester at the community college, Edith literally threw Allyson out of the house. Allyson had been dating a man at the time, and he assisted her in obtaining temporary housing while she was finishing school. When she finished the associate degree, she confronted Albert for the second time in her life.

Allyson went to her father's office at work and demanded that he cosign a $1,500 loan application. She told him it was the least he could do for all the sexual abuse she had put up with from him. He seemed to not quite understand what she meant, but he signed without hesitation. Allyson used this modest sum to get established in her own apartment. She worked full time while attending college for her baccalaureate degree. Recognized as an outstanding student, Allyson received a modest scholarship to help with tuition costs; however, the costs at the private university were high. Three years later when Allyson graduated with honors, Edith and Albert initiated an argument over how they supported her college studies. They attended graduation ceremonies and managed to spoil the day. "They came to the graduation, but wouldn't speak to me."

Allyson's marriage had taken place while she was working full time and studying for the baccalaureate degree. She told Ryan about the incest when their relationship became more serious than casual dating. From the moment she disclosed to him, he has been consistently supportive. Although it is difficult for him, he respects Allyson's decision to continue to include her parents in family functions. The wedding itself was grand. The hundred-plus guests in attendance would remember it as a storybook wedding. Allyson remembers the pain of being stranded in New York City after her mother physically pushed her out of the car. The pair had traveled into the city for gown shopping. When Allyson apologized for not being able to take Edith out for lunch because she had only $1.00 (she and Ryan paid for the wedding), Edith pushed her out from the car and left. The perfect mother–daughter outing was obviously supposed to have included lunch. There is perhaps some sort of strange irony that the official pictures of this storybook wedding would never be; Albert, assisting the professional photographer, failed to put the film in the camera.

Two years after her marriage, Allyson gave birth to Ryan Jr. The postpartum period was difficult for Allyson, who worried that she might become an abusive parent. There were no incidents to warrant this fear; she was, however, well aware of her parental role models. She made Ryan Sr. promise to watch closely and "never, never let anything happen to the baby." Allyson entered counseling during this time for depression. She was treated briefly with antidepressant medication and continued individual therapy for almost 1 year.

When I was younger, I thought that when I figured it all out, when I got to this point in my life—what I knew would be this point in my life— that I'd marry, I'd have a pretty wedding and children, that it would be okay. But I didn't anticipate that it would all come with me, and it would be a part of my everyday life. Somewhere back there it would always touch me.

There were some difficult times with Edith and Albert as Allyson began her own family. Because she very much values being a moral person and doing the right thing, Allyson does not want to deny her parents the right to their grandchild. However, she will never allow them to be alone with the child. The protection of her child is paramount to her. Her concerns appear justified.

Whenever our backs are turned, she [Edith] tries to take him, but we [Ryan Sr. and I] never leave my parents alone with the baby. One time Edith was changing his diaper; she'd be wiping him with a cloth and she'd say, "Oh! You really like it when I touch you there." I said, "You're making him clean and dry," you know, and it just made me upset.

There are days when Allyson feels that she just cannot cope. Talking to her counselor and her husband was helpful in validating her competencies as a new mother. Her value as a human being often needs reinforcement; Ryan Sr. meets this need. Her professional competency is obvious—to almost everyone but Allyson. Shortly before the interviews for this life history study began, Allyson was approached by an executive placement firm to interview for a prestigious position. The position was one that a professional with many more years of experience than Allyson would be eager to obtain. She was offered the position, and she accepted it. It was an outstanding accomplishment. During this time of celebration and stress—relocation would be necessary almost immediately—her parents made light of the accomplishment and sent more "hate mail," accusing Allyson of depriving them of their rightful "Grammy experience." In between life history interview #1 and #2, Allyson responded to Albert and Edith by writing the most direct communication she has had with them. In the last interview for this study, Allyson summed things up thus:

The bottom line is that if I had to do it over again I would wish they never had me. Truly . . . . You can make moments good, you can find peace and happiness sometimes, but the pain and the loss . . . I wish that they just didn't have me . . . . It's not really a life, because you're always waiting to die. You're always waiting for when your life is going to be over and then there's no more pain . . . I wish they didn't have me, and then maybe they would have been better to my sister. The only thing I can say about that is that if they didn't have me, maybe they would have really abused my sister worse, you know? Then I would wish they didn't have her either.

Key Informant #2: Becky

Becky is a 36-year-old White woman of Welsh descent. Her parents are Methodists; she is an active member of the Baptist church. Her father, the son of a Methodist minister, is a college graduate and president of a family-owned corporation. Her mother, born and raised in the midwestern United States and a high school graduate, is a school crossing guard. Married for 16 years, Becky has three children aged 13, 11, and 7. After completing 2 years at a state college, Becky left school to get married. She worked her way up to a managerial position in a clothing business, a position she left just prior to her first child's birth. She currently works part-time, organizing church youth group activities. Her husband, a barely literate high school graduate, works the night shift in a convenience store. She presents an overall wholesome appearance; minimal makeup is used, and her dark blond hair is pulled back at the neck. She has large green eyes and an energetic smile.

Becky is the third of four daughters. When Becky was 6 years old, the family moved to the Jersey Shore area from a neighboring state. The family remained in this home for the rest of her childhood. When I asked Becky if she remembered her original home, I did not fully realize the importance of my question. It was in that house that for the first 6 years of her life she reports she was repeatedly subjected to sexual abuse by her father.

More than the home itself, I remember things that happened in the home.

Although the sisters were close in age, the first three being each 2 years apart and the youngest being born 4 years after her, it was a solitary existence for Becky.

We were not allowed to be around other people, other children. We were kept separate. My two older sisters would go off to school and that would leave me at home.

Becky's mother did not work outside of the home. The days were spent in solitary play, watching her mother clean the house.

My memories are always of being alone. My mother also had no friends. No one ever came into the house. I guess what you would call the good memories: my mother would be cleaning the house; like she'd scrub the kitchen floor, and she'd move all the chairs into the living room, and I'd line them up—and cowboy shows were my favorite—and I'd line them up and ride stagecoach.

The neighborhood was actually built for low-income families. The houses were small, starter-type homes. Although there were many children, dolls, and bikes in the surrounding homes, Becky and her sisters were not part of that experience.

A few times children would come into the yard, but that's as far as they ever got. They were *never ever* permitted into the house, and even to come into the yard was rare. They were just asked to leave . . . . We didn't ask why. You just did what you were told, and you don't ask, you don't ask anything, and you don't have a say in anything.

When her sisters returned from school at the end of the day, they watched television or went to the room they shared; Becky had her own room. There was never any discussion in the house, even among the children. On a daily basis, actually several times a day, Becky's father would deliver a tirade over anything or nothing. The yelling was aggressive, abusive, and loud enough to be heard by the neighborhood. Becky never knew what the neighbors thought about this, because no interaction was allowed with neighbors. Becky recalls very clearly that the rules were, "You don't ask questions. You don't talk about the family or family business. You don't ever cry." In retrospect, she does not remember realizing that she was being abused. Indeed, she did not even remember the sexual abuse for almost 30 years. When the memories came, for Becky they made up for all the words never spoken. The memories came in pictures, and if ever it were the case, these pictures were worth a thousand words.

I see myself and I am very little . . . and that always happened at night.

At the urging of her therapists, Becky made the sketches shortly after she disclosed the incest. The baby/child curled in the crib-like bed radiates tension and fear; her father lurks in the doorway and then enters. Several years later, during her adolescence, Becky wrote descriptions of the actual sexual abuse in abstract poetry. She saved these writings, never really understanding them, but understanding that what was contained within the verse was very, very important; she just didn't know what it was. And for her, you don't ask.

Shortly before the family moved, the children were told to start getting their belongings ready. There had been no discussions about the move and no house-hunting trips. It was just done.

The new house was frightening. It was big and very old. There was a big upstairs and a big attic, and it was real creepy. It was like 150 years old and very scary . . . you didn't let it be known that you were scared.

There was a winding staircase to the second floor. Becky was assigned a room with her younger sister. The older girls also shared a room. All the bedrooms were on the same floor. The fourth bedroom was designated as the playroom.

Of course we never played there. That's where the games were kept.

There were many other new things that accompanied the move, many of them as frightening as the house itself. The family moved in July, and in September, Becky started school.

My mother never told me what school was about. I had no idea what was expected of me, what was going to happen, what they were going to do with me. I just did not know. And I'd never, *ever* been away from home. The only time I'd been away from home was when we'd all go grocery shopping together. So I had no connection with anything outside of my house.

Even though Becky was the third child in the family to enter school, the whole concept of school was a mystery to her. Her sisters never told her anything about it; homework was never discussed. Everyone lived his or her own little existence. There would be little change in this pattern over time; 10 years later, when Becky started college at her sister's alma mater, Becky knew little or nothing about college nor were her sister's experiences told— including the rape.

Many painful lessons were learned in school environments. In her first grade, Becky cried every day for the first month. She was in a classroom with children who talked to each other, laughed and played together after school, and asked questions. Becky was scared; she did not know how to do any of these things.

> I guess what finally got me to stop crying was—and I remember this so clearly—one day I was sitting in school and I was crying, and the teacher took me and locked me into the coat closet in the dark and she said to me, "Now, big girls don't cry, and if you cry you are going to be a bad girl." And I remember sitting there in the dark crying, but I swore that I was never, ever going to cry again. And I felt that was right, because that was the very thing that my parents always taught me: you don't cry absolutely you don't cry.

Her first venture into the world outside her family, her first grade, confirmed what she had always been taught: Don't ask and don't cry. Bad things are things that just have to be incorporated into everyday life. Her childhood was solitary and sad. She remembers thinking that it was strange that she was sad. After all, she had everything she needed; her parents told her that.

> We never asked for anything; you didn't do that. If there was a school project, you just made do . . . . My mother made most of our clothes; I got my sisters' old clothes . . . I decided to "get big" when I was in about seventh grade: I ate a lot to do this. It never occurred to me that I'd get fat. I just wanted to be bigger. Every Easter we got new dresses. We were taken to the store and told what we could have.

Easter was the same year after year. Every holiday was the same year after year: Get dressed up, go to church, and look like the best family. That was just what was done. Each of the children got a gift at Christmas. Becky describes Christmas as a very orderly ordeal. Each child would, in turn, open his or her gift. The girls did not give gifts to each other; they did not talk to each other. There was no money to buy gifts even if they had thought about it. At age 16, each child began working at McDonald's. All earnings were put into the bank for college. The girls worked full time at McDonald's every summer. Because they were so close in age, it happened that they were working at the same time. Being in a different environment did not change their pattern of noninteraction.

> You were supposed to work. You were supposed to be the best worker. It was the same if I worked with my sisters or anyone else; I was there to work.

Not only holidays but also every day was predictable. Breakfast was eaten in the kitchen every day except Sunday. Sunday breakfast and every supper except Saturday night supper were eaten in the dining room. Becky's mother did all the cooking except on Saturday morning when her father always made breakfast. There was never any deviation from this pattern.

> *Once,* when we were much older, my sisters were already in college, we [the children], joked among ourselves about who was going to ask Dad to buy pizza that night. Of course we didn't do this in front of him.

When Becky told me about the pizza discussion, I questioned her as to the outcome, that is, who finally did ask Dad for pizza. "No one. You never, ever ask."

In addition to working to save money for college—Becky did not want to go to college but that was not her decision to make—she kept herself occupied during her teenage years with sports. Her father had decided that she would participate in the township softball league; she later added field hockey to her schedule. Becky was a gifted athlete; she excelled in sports. She remembers waiting and waiting to hear *her father* say she was good. But acknowledgments were not to be. Her mother, as well as all the coaches, noticed her ability. But she wanted her father's approval.

> It didn't matter what Mom said because we knew that didn't count. Dad was the one who knew everything; he could do everything. We always knew that. He told us we weren't musical, for example. So that was that. It was his approval that counted. He had a way, though, of turning everything around so that anything good was because of him; *we* were never good enough. He dished out approval backhandedly. For instance, when I went for my driver's test and scored 100. I didn't make one mistake. I came out and was feeling at the top of the world, and my father said, "Oh, of course you did; I had the air-conditioning on for him, he would have given you 100 no matter what!" Just in all those little subtle ways he took the credit. It was something he did. And that's why you got what you got.

Township sport teams participate in many activities in addition to practice and games. Becky remembers the first time the team was to go away for a week of hockey camp.

> I couldn't ask him. You don't ask. So I told him that the coach wanted me to do this because I was the team captain. He [father] had to make sure that it wasn't my decision. I never, ever was allowed to decide these things.

High school graduation was not particularly memorable. "We came home and had cake. I got a check for graduation—everyone got a check for graduation—I never saw it." The graduation check went into the bank for the college education that Becky did not want.

> It was just told that you were going [college]. We didn't even fill out the applications. It was all done by Father. He had complete control of everything.

She entered the state college as a liberal arts major. Becky is very appreciative of the girls in her dormitory who were outgoing and kind and sought out even the quiet girls to join in activities and be part of the group. She learned to laugh and to make small talk. If they had not approached her in friendship, she would not have had any idea what to do or what was expected of her.

> The girls on my floor in the dorm were my saving grace; they really were, and once I got used to being there, it had an incredibly freeing feeling. It was like there was a load lifted off my mind; there was a cloud that was lifted. Just being free of my father's yelling and carrying on. It was like there was always a cloud over the house.

Becky worked on campus. She never saw a paycheck; all pay went directly home to the bank. She no longer had hand-me-down clothes; that had stopped when she "got bigger" than her sisters. Becky stayed at the college on weekends; this was different from what her sister had done, but Becky knew she did not want to go back. She was beginning to feel bigger and stronger as a person. The only other good educational experience she had had previously was in the fifth grade. That was the year of her favorite teacher; Mrs. White made Becky feel special.

> I was her favorite. She picked me to clean the boards, smiled at me . . . she was kind to me . . . I didn't know what to say to her; I never said anything . . . I didn't know there was anything to say.

In college, Becky was learning about how people do things. She was considering majoring in psychology, but her college career ended before that became a reality. In the October of her sophomore year, she was raped by a man she had met at the church near the campus. She went into the college chapel immediately after being raped. She sat there and cried. A girl she had known since her second grade came into the chapel. Becky tried to tell her what had happened, but the girl would not believe her. Becky found this reaction to her disclosure devastating. She sat alone in the college campus and understood, because she had been taught well, that "If something bad happens, that's a secret."

> That was the final straw for me. That was what said: "Don't ever trust anyone. It's just not worth it. You make enemies that way. You lose friends that way. Be whatever it is that people want you to be, and then they'll like you." That just confirmed all that for me.

Events moved quickly after she was raped. Becky, who was just beginning to get a sense of life outside of her home, no longer felt that she belonged in college. She had loved living in the school dormitory. For the first time, she got a close-up view of how 'real people' lived. She saw what small talk was all about. She spent many of her childhood years wondering what people talked about. She had been captain of the town's softball team, but she had never really been part of the team.

> After practice, I'd see the girls walking together off the field talking and laughing, and I never knew why they would do that. I knew that we were there to practice. We were there to listen to the coaches train us to be the best . . . I thought it was very strange that they would have anything to say to each other, let alone to the coaches, after practice.

After the rape, she felt that she was no longer part of the college scene. She agonized over what she was to do. But in truth she felt that she had no choice. So she retreated to familiar behaviors: being whatever people wanted her to be. John, the rapist, wanted a wife. Becky, his virgin victim, would comply.

Becky had met John in September; he raped her in October, and in December she told her parents that at the end of the school year she would be marrying John. This was not what she was "supposed" to do; her father had decided that all the children were to go to college. The family's financial support was withdrawn at the end of the year—married daughters do not go to college. Becky worked all summer at McDonald's to pay for the wedding. Her sisters never discussed the wedding with Becky. John was from a large, traditional Italian family that "expected" the usual church wedding and reception. The entire wedding was Becky's responsibility. Becky's wedding would be a first in several ways, not the least of which was that it would be her first: She had "never, ever" even been to a wedding. The day of her wedding, as she stood at the back door of the church on her father's arm, she clearly remembers not wanting to get married.

> I wanted to go, to get out of there, but I didn't know how; I didn't know how to make decisions. I was so sad. I was very upset standing there. My father said, "Stop crying!"

The marriage initiated a pattern that was to persist for years: Everything was Becky's responsibility, for example, the upkeep of the home—both inside and outside—the care of the children, and anything that was required to make John's life easier. Years later, after the incest memories came and after her suicide attempts, and following therapy, Becky asked her husband about that night in college when he raped her. He laughed. He didn't think it was rape; he thought it was his right. There had been a man like this in her life before; she called him Dad.

For the first 13 years of her marriage, Becky did what she had been taught so well: work hard, be the best, don't ask questions, and don't cry. Only rarely did she deviate from the rules; one such occasion was shortly after the birth of her first child. It was the middle of the night, and the baby was sick with a high fever. She was trying to quiet the baby, as her husband did not want his sleep disturbed. After several hours, out of sheer exhaustion and worry, Becky began to cry. John entered the room, looked at Becky, and said, "Are you crying?" Without waiting for an answer, he began to laugh and went back to bed. Becky resolved anew never to cry again. Her resolve lasted several years.

She reports feeling unhappy and trapped. Her minister had for some time been encouraging her to seek counseling. "I finally agreed just because I was so tired . . . I was always taking care of everybody else." Many sessions into counseling, she disclosed the rape, but she did not call it rape. "I just told him [the counselor] what happened. He said, 'Becky, you was raped.'" The counselor immediately referred Becky to the Rape Crisis Center, as he did not have expertise in that area. Becky is extremely grateful for that referral. The Rape Crisis Center, located in the YWCA, is staffed by a group of "exceptionally patient and caring therapists." Becky reports feeling very safe at the YWCA; she also recalls that from the very beginning she wanted to learn how to say things—even though she did not know what it was that she wanted to say. Talking, however, was not without guilt. The guilt proved to be overwhelming; Becky suffered a major depressive episode with suicidal ideation, and although hospitalization was recommended, Becky only agreed to spend some time with friends from the church who offered her their home. Becky reports:

[I was] confused, depressed, hopeless for about three months . . . then I started having flashbacks. Of course, at the time I didn't know what they were. I called my therapist. She told me to come right in [to the office]. I saw scenes in my mind, but I felt like I was right there. She told me to draw them. It was my father coming into my room. I was very small.

Becky's support system during this time was made up of her church friends; in addition, she and her husband were seeing a family counselor at the church. Because they had been there for her throughout her recent depression and attempted suicide, Becky disclosed the incest when they asked how she was doing. The friends hugged her and stated their willingness to "help in any way." The counselor cautioned her not to disclose to her husband.

He [the counselor] knew John laughed when I tried to talk to him about the rape. The counselor didn't think that John could be trusted with this; I would just get hurt.

Becky's disclosures, which came more than 30 years after the incest began, came in succession: to therapists, church friends, counselors. Becky's immediate reaction to disclosing was a disinterest in seeing or talking to her parents, especially her father.

I feel guilty talking about it; like I'm doing something bad. I thought if I saw him, somehow he would know that I told, and you're not supposed to talk. There's no need to. But I'm learning that I need to . . . I need to do this for me . . .

THEMES AND SUBTHEMES

Four themes emerged from the data: (a) coping, (b) self-image, (c) communication barriers, and (d) communication facilitators. In addition, eight subthemes were identified: eating disturbances, sports activities, boundaries, rigidity, phoniness, moral values, protectiveness, and spirituality. Although the themes were often concurrent, sequential, and interrelated, for presentation purposes the four major themes are discussed separately.

The overall framework for the conduct of this life history study was the disclosure of incest. Therefore, each of the twelve themes that emerged contributes to the composite picture of the cultural context in which the incest and disclosure took place. Each theme is discussed here, and brief quotations, which were selected from the data set because of their recurrence in interviews, are given as examples. Because of the abbreviation of the dissertation for the chapter, only a few examples are given in this section.

Theme #1: Coping

Often incest survivors criticize themselves for the ways in which they coped; it may be difficult to admit some of the things that had to be done in order to survive. The range of coping behaviors is vast, from highly perfected distraction techniques to more complex dissociative disorders, including multiple personality disorder. In this study, subconcepts of coping that emerged were eating disorders, involvement in sports, and spirituality.

Becky dissociated herself from the incest for 30 years. Some degree of dissociation as a common response to incest is now well recognized by therapists. Courtois (1988) notes that Summit (1983) and Shengold (1979) discussed splitting as a coping mechanism, as did Brickman (1984) who identified a range of dissociative behaviors that she termed "sliding personality." The very mechanisms employed for coping may give rise to other issues. For example, Brickman's continuum of personalities may be associated with a survivor feeling like a "phony": Key Informant #1, Allyson, stated, "One minute I'm a competent professional and then I'm suicidal, Who am I really?"

Elaborated Description

Allyson recalls coping with abuse on an everyday basis while growing up. What surprises her is that coping is *still* very much a part of her life. Coping with the memories of the abuse is half of the picture; coping with the memories of what she had to do to survive is the other half. For example, the subtheme "eating disorder" was a big part of her life.

> I'll be in line at the checkout counter and see a young girl with three boxes of laxatives, and I know. And I wonder how I looked back then . . . it was a very hard time. I was very much into my eating disorder; I was bulimic. It's very painful to think about that time.

Elaborated Description

The mechanism that was used for coping—having control in one area of her life—escalated to the degree that, even today, excessive diet control and exercising manifest, especially in times of increased stress. It is significant to note that Allyson's eating disorder served as a coping attempt in several ways. On a daily basis, it gave her a sense of control, and in the long range, it was the symptom that brought her to a counselor for the first time. In addition, it was the resultant weakening in her state of health that tired her to the point that she gave up keeping secrets and disclosed to her best friend.

> I understand a lot of people who do that [change their name] have this kind of history. They have to change their names and do things like that. I can say I just hated my name. You know, but it was nice . . . cause a separate identity came along with it.

Elaborated Description

Becky spent much of her childhood coping with feelings that did not have names. She knew she was sad, but she did not know why or what was driving her. "I ran on the field." When she trained for sports, she trained extremely hard; she would run 5 or 6 miles before practice, and she would continue running after practice.

Theme #2: Self-Image

The second major theme was self-image, with subconcepts of phoniness and being a moral person. Self-esteem is a basic issue for women. When children are deprived of the opportunity to feel good about themselves and have no sense of being precious and valued just because they exist—separate from anything they do—the damage is done at a core level. Accomplishments gained seem to the survivor to be undeserved. Survivors from many different backgrounds seem to share one quality rather consistently, that of low self-esteem. Persistent feelings of being bad, contaminated, or unworthy are intricately connected with other "self" words that may be used to describe the adult survivor: self-effacing and self-depreciating. Self-esteem is experienced in the moment; there are fluctuations, depending on the circumstances and the stressors of the situation. For survivors, these fluctuations can be rapid and continual. For Allyson and Becky, self-image had something to do with being a fraud/phony or being a moral person; it had everything to do with never being good enough.

Elaborated Description

Although Becky's mother would, at times, comment on how well Becky had done, it meant nothing, because the only person who counted, the only person who "knew everything" was her father. This was reinforced by people outside the family as well. Becky's father was a leader in the church and a college-educated businessman. It was, however, he himself who most often stressed his perfection.

> I don't feel like I have a legitimate reason to feel so bad . . . and I say to myself, "What the hell do I have to feel so bad about? My parents did not lock me in the closet. My mother did not hang me by my hair in the garage." Why do I have to feel this bad?

Theme #3: Communication Barriers

From the perspective of family systems, incestuous families have been found to have rigid boundaries to the outside world. The typical incest family is socially, psychologically, and, often, physically isolated (Courtois, 1988). "Although incest occurs, it is largely denied and unacknowledged by all family members. This disconfirmation allows for its continuance while communicating to the victim that it is something that is not to be discussed" (Courtois, 1988, p. 46).

Elaborated Description

Throughout the interviews, both Allyson and Becky strongly associated talking with being bad. In Allyson's family, it might spoil the picture. In Becky's family, talking was a sign of weakness: "You can't handle everything yourself."

Theme #4: Communication Facilitators

An examination of the experiences and situations that facilitated communication in general and communication about incest in particular is presented in this section. While this theme was consistently labeled during inter-rater reliability checks, it was the least prevalent of the themes. The subtheme *protectiveness* was strongly associated with communication facilitation.

Elaborated Description

Allyson accuses herself of having been very naïve; however, she truly cannot recall hearing anyone discussing parents having sex with their children. Unlike her eating disorder, bulimia, which she would hear discussed on national talk shows several years later, incest was still not a "talk show" topic. The opportunity to hear incest being discussed triggered Allyson's awareness of wrongdoing in the family system. It was after this discussion in school that she states her "conscious life" began.

> I didn't do it [disclose to second oldest brother, Steve] for the right reasons. I didn't do it in order to help somebody else.

DISCUSSION

This study examined the self-reported steps taken by incest survivors when disclosing incest. In attempting to trace the steps taken by incest survivors, Part I of the study consisted of two life histories, and Part II was a survey by therapists who counsel survivors. The sequence of steps reported in the life histories was compared to the sequence of steps identified by therapists as being the most typically reported by survivors. In addition, both the life history data and the survey data are discussed in relation to the steps of the whistleblowing process reported by Stewart (1980).

Whistleblowing in Small Organizations

There is ever-increasing evidence that climates and cultures of organizations influence whistleblowing. In their review and analysis of studies that conceptualize and measure climate in different ways, Miceli and Near (1992) note that organizational climates that are less defensive and more participatory are associated with whistleblowing. The organization's environment plays a role in the decision to blow the whistle. In Allyson's family, this belief was especially evident. Allyson remembered very clearly thinking that the family would be destroyed if she told the secret. She feared that the children would be taken away, and the whole family would blame her. She was convinced that her role was to keep the family together. When she was ultimately confronted with the need to protect her younger sister, balancing protection of her sister with the protection of the family's survival became an agonizing decision for her.

Drawing from the literature on norm conformity, which suggests that the quality of the evidence showing wrongdoing will influence whistleblowing (Greenberger, Miceli, & Cohen, 1987), studies have shown (Miceli & Near, 1985) that more whistleblowing occurs where the evidence of the wrongdoing is clear and direct. The messages that abound in incestuous families are veiled in secrecy. Both life history informants doubted their intellectual abilities. Self-image emerged as a thematic category with self-deprecating remarks being prevalent in the case of both women. Even potential whistleblowers who are not hampered by these cognitive restraints must attend to analyzing the signals the organization has given regarding its likely response to whistleblowing behavior. Becky knew that "you never, ever ask questions" and that "you never, ever have a say in anything." Allyson was very clear that her role was to keep the family together. At one point or another, both informants voiced the questions: What would be the point [of disclosing]? What would be accomplished? The perception that an organization would respond to whistleblowing by correcting the wrongdoing is associated with greater whistleblowing by individual members (Miceli & Near, 1992). Organizational responsiveness was perceived by the informants in this study to be nonexistent, that is, no correction of any alleged wrongdoing would occur. Becky, of course, did not grapple with this decision until years after the abuse. However, she had always been taught that her father was perfect and that nothing he did was less than perfect.

Disclosure of Incest as Whistleblowing

Early in this study, the view of families as organizations was established. From this premise, it would have been expected that families would more closely resemble small organizations than large organizations. Although making such a determination was not a specific part of this study, the literature on whistleblowing has identified how the phenomenon manifests in organizations of different sizes. There is, however, no consensus on whistleblowing specific to the size of organizations. For example, although it was at first believed that there would be more internal whistleblowing in small organizations and more external whistleblowing in large organizations, studies do not support this pattern (Miceli & Near, 1985). When the wrongdoing is incest, the family seems to more closely resemble in organizational structure a large (that is, tall) organizations. For example, the distance between parties in the flow of communication is great in both large organizations and in incestuous families. In incestuous families, the distance may be accounted for by a void rather than a particular series of persons who might impede upward communication. Another point of similarity is the failure of top managers to directly encourage whistleblowing by making members aware of established channels to report wrongdoing. In tall organizations, this may be the result of the great distance between the top management and the workers. In families, the reason may be more self-protective. A last significant point is that unlike members of small organizations who may feel greater satisfaction than those in larger organizations and, therefore, choose to blow the whistle internally in the hope that this would be less damaging to the organization, the survivors in this study viewed internal whistleblowing as more damaging to the family than external whistleblowing. Allyson Kenny attributed little significance to the first time she disclosed to someone outside the family; it was an external disclosure and, therefore, was not a traumatic undertaking. However, she still remembers the disclosure to her brother with much guilt.

Organizations that are bureaucratic or authoritarian are less open to whistleblowing challenges (Weinstein, 1979). Becky's family was clearly authoritarian. In rigidly structured organizations in which a single view predominates, dissent is likely to be ignored (Schwenk, 1988). More than 30 years after the onset of the abuse, Becky's father dismissed her recollections as simply "wrong."

Dilemmas of Conducting Life History Research

Consistent with the life history method is the opportunity throughout the study for informant input and decision. For example, the actual setting for the interviews was a decision made by the informants. The decisions subsequently became part of the data. When Becky, without a moment's hesitation, elected to meet at the YWCA, the investigator noted this decision-making process. In the course of the interviews, it became clear that a *safe, respectful* environment was important to Becky not only for the research interviews but also for her initial incest disclosure. An antecedent to the disclosure process for Becky was involvement in an environment that gives high priority to communication. Becky participates in several discussion groups at the YWCA, including a class that teaches how to communicate in job interview situations. It was, therefore, from a methodological dilemma that data emerged, which the investigator may not have accessed otherwise.

Allyson Kenny's interviews were conducted at her college; the importance of this choice has already been presented. Because the college's significance to Allyson was clear early in the interviews, the investigator did not consider changing locations. After Allyson had moved out of the state, there were several telephone interviews and one longer interview in a hotel lobby. Although Allyson had been quite open in the early sessions, in this interview she was much more so. It is a dilemma for the investigator when considering alternative interview sites. The trade-offs include leaving a setting that seems to be conducive to productive interviewing for untried settings. The investigator can only speculate how altering Becky's interview settings would have affected the data. It is a trade-off that in retrospect would have been made.

It would have been impossible to collect data of such a sensitive nature without successfully establishing trust. Although building a trusting relationship is more appropriate to the discussion of a therapeutic relationship, a sense of being safe and respected had also to be established in this investigator–informant relationship. The ability to foster such a climate is clearly a prerequisite to the conduct of life history research. The dilemma inherent in creating such a climate is that should some information simply be ignored or is there an ethical responsibility inherent in fostering such a climate? The investigator used her training as a psychotherapist to clarify the information and direct the informant to share it with her therapist. For example, when Becky began an interview with the discussion of the nightmares/ night terrors that had begun during the previous week, anxiety-reducing intervention was needed, and it was provided. She was then encouraged to contact her therapist that day for an appointment. In addition, emergency strategies to deal with the terrors were given in the event that Becky was not able to reach her therapist before that night. This is not to say that only trained therapists should be open to discussion of emotionally charged issues. This investigator, lacking experience in the conduct of actual life history research, drew on the clinical competencies she brought to the situation. Nontherapist investigators who have experience with the method would use equally ethical interventions.

Clearly, these dilemmas give rise to interesting methodological issues. The deliberate use of multiple interview sites could be part of the methodology. A theoretical rationale supportive of this decision is specifically pertinent to this study and relates to memory. Memories can be triggered by environmental cues. A particular scent, a type of lighting, furniture, formality, or informality may influence the content and/or process of the informants, both of whom have been in psychotherapy, and as the investigator is a psychotherapist, it is an approach for use in future studies. The transcriptionist's selection followed the steps outlined in the methodology section of this study. Based on the events described, enhancement of this selection process is indicated. Specifically, the interventions used by the investigator with the replacement transcriptionist should be part of the original methodology.

Ethical Issues of Life History Research

Although all investigators who conduct research involving human subjects are bound by an ethical code of conduct, life history research gives rise to specific ethical issues. The impact of participating in life history research must be considered in relation to the informants, the researcher, and all others involved, for example, the transcriptionists.

Issues for consideration in relation to the informants include time frame: At what point is the study over? Both Allyson and Becky were highly committed to participating in the study to the best of their ability. Information was shared willingly, with a desire to contribute to the research. After the actual interviews were completed, there were several telephone contacts. Although achieving closure is usually valued in dealing with psychological material, the ethics of forced closure must be considered. Rather than imposing an arbitrary time limit for post-interview conversations, that is, a forced closure, this time period can be valuable for the afterlife of life history research. The importance of afterlife is recognized in the literature and discussed as a powerful mix of lives, text, and context. Afterlife is a recognition that the life history process continues beyond the crystallization of the narrative into text to include its impact on the lives of its narrator and investigator (Blackman, 1992). It is because of this scope of impact that the entire study must be conducted with close attention to ethical implications. The afterlife will eventually include not only the informants, investigator, and transcriptionists, but the readers as well.

An immediate impact on the investigator occurred after the first interview with Key Informant #1 and can best be described as an experience with comparative empathy. While driving home from the interview, the investigator experienced, in a way she had never felt during 19 years as a psychotherapist, the pain of the events presented in the interview. The investigator, known by her clients and peers to be an empathic listener, was not surprised by the content of the interview, because she had had extensive experience with survivors. What was different and surprising was the impact of hearing the story without the protection of a professional relationship. When a therapist is working with a survivor, there is the knowledge that the therapist can help; knowing that there was no such goal-directed plan removed that protection. Clearly, protectiveness is a phenomenon in need of further exploration in families, in therapeutic relationships, and in life history methodology. Protectiveness emerged as a subtheme for both communication barriers and communication facilitators. Additionally, the therapists surveyed commented on their former clients sensing that the therapists needed to be protected from the pain of hearing about incest.

The knowledge that life history research has an afterlife poses additional ethical issues for publication decisions. Key informants who give informed consent to participate in a study may not consider post-study publication and afterlife issues. The investigator discussed this with Allyson and Becky. Both informants were willing and eager to have the research responsibly disseminated.

Policy Recommendations

Current approaches to child abuse detection and prevention make some serious assumptions. "Go. Run. Tell," "Just Say No," "Good Touch and Bad Touch": These are catch phrases used in educational programs on child abuse. The phrases are simple enough but require skills for their communication. The acquisition of basic communication skills must be addressed. In addition, decision-making skills are inherent in the techniques currently being taught. For example, *is* it good touch or bad touch?

Decision making is not something that is encouraged in authoritarian families; being a competent decision maker is not part of a survivor's self-image. Both Allyson and Becky shared an important communication skill that was never fully directed: writing. Allyson's term paper on incest was carefully read and approved by the faculty, but her words were never given a voice. Becky wrote poetry but no one read it. Both women knew that what they were writing meant something, but, lacking confidence in themselves, they thought it could not *really* be important. Clinicians value and use clients' writing in treatment; this was specifically emphasized by Bass (Bass & Davis, 1988) who is not a therapist but a writing teacher. Early use of this communication skill, written expression, should be included in detection and prevention programming. Becky "treasured" little scraps of paper she carried in her pockets, with words, ideas, and stories scribbled on them. She did not know how to orally communicate these things; indeed, she did not even know one could.

Alternative Perspectives on Disclosure

The data from survivors and therapists reported in this study provided a framework for new perspectives on disclosure. The sequence of steps in the disclosure of incest can now be viewed from an insider's perspective. A requisite to description of the context of disclosure is an understanding and appreciation of the context of incest. The structure and functioning of the family was evident in the details presented in the life history. The behaviors that facilitated the persistence of wrongdoing form the backdrop when we view the event of disclosure. The themes of self-image, coping, and communication barriers are the fiber of the backdrop. The subtheme, *protectiveness*, served as an antecedent to the disclosure, while at the same time it was part of the context of nondisclosure. The survey data (not reported here) suggest that this protectiveness may extend to the therapist as well. Several respondents included notes suggesting that they may have treated many more incest survivors than they realize; in retrospect, they think the clients may have tried to communicate this.

Limitations

Although the investigator is an experienced therapist, she had never conducted life history research. This limitation was minimized by ongoing consultation with the methodologist on the dissertation committee. Consultation occurred throughout the study and increased as the data were collected and analyzed.

Audiotaping may have initially inhibited the free flow of conversation; however, this limitation was minimized by explaining to the informant the purpose of the taping, the disposition of the actual tape, and the option of stopping the interview at any time without consequence. As had been expected, both key informants seemed to forget about the taping a few minutes into the interview.

Directions for Further Research

Policy recommendations need to be studied further. If communication skills and opportunity to speak are antecedents to disclosure, the methods of providing these skills and opportunities need to be developed.

Significant people in the lives of survivors need to be studied. For example, athletic coaches may be in a position to provide a description of disclosure attempts. In addition, writing teachers and therapists need an increased awareness of the context required for disclosure to occur.

The whistleblowing literature has identified that there is a greater likelihood of whistleblowing when the effects of the wrongdoing spread to harm increased numbers of people. This study, with its strong protectiveness theme, tends to support that; however, whistleblowing in incestuous families has not been studied from the perspective of a member of the organization who is *not* the victim.

The perceived importance of internal versus external whistleblowing must be further clarified for a more detailed explanation of the two processes. From these suggested studies will come the data necessary for prediction of circumstances that can encourage potential whistleblowers.

SUMMARY

Watson and Watson-Franke (1985) note that there are key questions that can be addressed at the conclusion of a study in which the investigator is used as an instrument. Two of these questions are as follows: (a) What information is volunteered and what is given in response to direct questioning? (b) How does the investigator motivate the informant to relate her life history? Whereas these questions have been dealt with in the methodology section of this study, at this point, a more comprehensive response is possible—comprehensive in that the findings of this study constitute the answer to these questions and the answers to the research questions posed. Both the investigator–informant relationship and the conduct of the interviews reflected themes of importance to the informants. The themes that emerged from the life history data—coping, self-image, communication barriers, and communication facilitators—tell us about the content, context, antecedents, and sequelae of incest disclosure. Additionally, in retrospect, it can be seen that these themes made possible the volunteering of information, the answering of direct questions, and the motivation to relate life histories. The method is respectful of the informant, thereby protecting her self-esteem. Safeguards were included in the design to enable the informant to cope with the emotionally intense data. The use of the investigator as an instrument provided ongoing facilitation of communication and the opportunity to deal with any actual or perceived barriers to communication. Although the complexity of the data and the data collection process were considerable, the principles that guided the process are basic to the fostering of communication. The informants in this study were repeatedly appreciative of the opportunity to tell their story. Both Allyson and Becky carefully reviewed interview data, providing clarification, corrections, and validity. Long after the last interviews were conducted, Becky sent the following reflections on the themes that emerged from the data.

Theme #1: Coping

Eating is one, if not the only, thing I feel like I have control of. It's something that everyone else says I have to do but they can't make me. I've had other things forced on me but not this. I have had so many people telling me what I have to do in my life, this is my way of saying I've had enough. I'll do what I want to do; I'll look like I want to look. I'll disappear and there is nothing you can do to stop me. The more you don't like the fact that I starve myself the more I will do it.

I tried your way. I ate a lot at one time to make you happy. I wanted to be big so you'd like me, but it never worked. You just made more fun of me. I wasn't good enough. Now I'm doing things my way and you can say whatever you will, but I'm not listening. Eating anything is too much because I don't want your approval anymore. I'll do what I damn well please.

Theme #2: Self-Image

I have spent my life doing what is right, being good, being pure. Ironically, all hell was breaking loose around me in my home as I was growing up. But it was wrong to swear, it was wrong to drink, it was wrong to talk about family secrets. Now it seems like all of these are all that I can do. I swear a lot, I drink wine every night to take the edge off life, and the family secrets are coming out one by one. I experienced a lot of guilt at first whenever any of these happened. Now I feel it is just one more way to express my freedom. I will do whatever is in me that wants to come out. Even in participating in this life [life history study] I am being bad because I am saying things about the family that were supposed to be kept a secret. I won't allow the old guilt to control me any longer.

Themes #3 and 4: Communication Barriers/Facilitators

I feel such a loss as I think back on my childhood. How different it could have been if I just had someone to talk to. And now it is still so strange to express my feelings. I don't know how to think for myself. In my childhood it worked because we went to our father for everything.

But now who do I go to, how do I give myself permission to make decisions for myself? I always feel as if I'm supposed to run to somebody else for the answers.

As a child, not holding personal conversations with people kept me away from others, that's what my father wanted. But now I find personal conversations awkward and uncomfortable, but I want them desperately. It is a wall I keep chipping away at.

Allyson, at the conclusion of the study, encouraged the investigator to make the research available to many professionals so that it would be "read and heard." She shared the following entry from her diary:

... it takes the objective eye of many to find the truth. My pages become full and yet remain empty in that they are unshared.

This chapter is an attempt to honor that wish.

NOTE

1. The procedures detailed in the preceding paragraphs were followed for the analysis of the life history data. However, an alternative method of data organization and analysis was developed by the investigator during the course of the study and has been termed "Multichromatic Analysis Technique" (MAT). MAT replaces the use of cumbersome index cards and marking pens. It is the investigator's belief that this newer technique is an example of the diffusion of innovation—plastic-coated, colored paper clips. The steps in the process are as follows: (a) Place typed interview transcripts in a binder. (b) Read through the interviews, making light pencil checkmarks in margins where data appear to be a potential theme. (c) Arrange several piles of colored paper clips. (d) Reread interviews, attaching a paper clip to the right-hand edge of the page, marking a particular quotation that appears to represent a theme; use a different colored clip for each theme. (e) Reread numerous times, changing the theme category of any quotation by replacing the clip with one of a different color. (f) Give the binder, with clips attached, to a reviewer. (g) As the reviewer reads the quotations, she or he attaches a different colored clip *to* the existing clip whenever she or he does not agree with the theme category to which the quotation has been assigned. (h) Discuss until agreement is reached, changing assignments as necessary. MAT offers the advantage of keeping all the data together so that information is not accidentally misplaced, as is the risk when using individual cards.

REFERENCES

Aberle, D. F. (1967). The psychosocial analysis of a Hopi life history. In R. Hunt (Ed.), *Personalities and culture* (pp. 79–138). New York, NY: Natural History Press.

Alexander, J. G., de Chesnay, M., Marshall, E., Campbell, A. R., Johnson, S., & Wright, R. (1989). Research note: Parallel reactions in rape victims and rape researchers. *Violence and Victims, 4*(1), 57–62.

Ammon-Gaberson, K. B., & Piantanida, M. (1988). Generating results from qualitative data. *Image, 20*(3),159–161.

Anderson, R. E., & Carter, I. (1984). *Human behavior in the social environment: A social systems approach* (3rd ed.). New York, NY: Aldine.

Bass, E., & Davis, L. (1988). *The courage to heal.* New York, NY: Harper & Row.

Blackman, M. B. (1992). The afterlife of the life history [Editorial]. *Journal of Narrative and Life History, 2*(1), 1–9.

Brickman, J. (1984). Feminist, nonsexist, and traditional models of therapy: Implications for working with incest. *Women and Therapy, 3*(1), 49–67.

Carter, E., & McGoldrick, M. (1980). *The family life: A framework for family therapy.* New York, NY: Gardner Press.

Courtois, C. A. (1988). *Healing the incest wound.* New York, NY: W. W. Norton.

de Chesnay, M. (1985). Father-daughter incest: An overview. *Behavioral Sciences and the Law, 3*(4), 391–402.

de Chesnay, M. (1991, March 13–15). *Cartharsis as an outcome of naturalistic research.* Paper presented on ethics panel at the annual meeting of the Society for Applied Anthropology, Charleston, NC.

Dobbert, M. C. (1982). *Ethnographic research.* New York, NY: Praeger.

Dollard, J. (1935). *Criteria for the life history, with analysis of six notable documents.* New York, NY: P. Smith.

Etizoni, A. (1964). *Modern organizations.* Englewood Cliffs, NJ: Prentice-Hall.

Field, P. A., & Morse, J. M. (1985). *Nursing research: The application of qualitative approaches.* Rockville, MD: Aspen.

Finkelhor, D. (1984). *Child sexual abuse: New theory and research.* New York, NY: The Free Press.

Gelles, R., & Pedrick, C. (1985). *Intimate violence in families.* Beverly Hills, CA: Sage.

Glazer, M. P., & Glazer, P. M. (1989).*Whistleblowers.* New York, NY: Basic Books.

Greenberger, D. B., Miceli, M. P., & Cohen, D. (1987). Oppositionists and group norms: The reciprocal influence of whistleblowers and coworkers. *Journal of Business Ethics, 7*, 527–542.

Hughes, C. C. (1965). The life history in cross-cultural psychiatric research. In J. M. Murphy & A. H. Leighton (Eds.), *Approaches to cross-cultural psychiatry* (pp. 285–328). Ithaca, NY: Cornell University Press.

Hughes, C. C. (1974). *Eskimo boyhood: An autobiography in psychosocial perspective.* Lexington, KY: University of Kentucky Press.

Kardiner, A. (1945). *The psychological frontiers of society.* New York, NY: Columbia University Press.

Kluckhohn, C. (1943). Review of Sun chief: The autobiography of a Hopi Indian, L. W. Simmons (Ed.). *American Anthropologist, 45,* 267–270.

Langness, L. L., & Frank, G. (1981). *Lives: An anthropological approach to biography.* Novato, CA: Chandler & Sharp.

Lincoln, Y., & Guba, E. (1985). *Naturalistic inquiry.* Newbury Park, CA: Sage.

Miceli, M., & Near, J. P. (1985). Characteristics of organizational climate and perceived wrongdoing associated with whistleblowing decisions. *Personnel Psychology, 38,* 525–544.

Miceli, M., & Near, J. P. (1992). *Blowing the whistle.* New York, NY: Macmillan.

Miles, M. B., & Huberman, A. M. (1984). *Qualitative data analysis: A sourcebook of new methods.* Beverly Hills, CA: Sage.

Miller, A. (1989). *For your own good.* Toronto, Canada: Collins.

Parsons, T. (1964). *Social structure and personality.* New York, NY: The Free Press.

Radin, P. (1920). The autobiography of a Winnebago Indian. *University of California Publications in American Archaeology and Ethnology, 16,* 381–473.

Sapir, E. (1934). The emergence of the concept of personality in a study of culture. *Journal of Social Psychology, 5,* 408–415.

Schwenk, C. (1988). *The essence of decision making.* Lexington, MA: Lexington Books.

Shengold, L. (1979). Child abuse and deprivation: Soul murder. *Journal of the American Psychoanalytic Association, 27,* 533–559.

Simmons, L., (Ed.). (1942). *Sun chief: The autobiography of a Hopi Indian.* New Haven, CT: Yale University Press.

Spradley, J. P. (Ed.). (1969). *Guests never leave hungry: The autobiography of James Sewid, a Kwakiutl Indian.* New Haven, CT: Yale University Press.

Stewart, L. (1980). Whistleblowing: Implications for organizational communication. *Journal of Communication, 30*(4), 90–101.

Summit, R. (1983). The child sexual abuse accommodation syndrome. *Child Abuse and Neglect, 7,* 177–193.

Thomas, W. I., & Znaniecki, F. (1920–1927). *The Polish peasant in Europe and America* (Vols. 1 and 2). New York, NY: Alfred A. Knopf.

Walters, K. D. (1975). Your employees' right to blow the whistle. *Harvard Business Review, 53*(4), 26–34.

Watson, L. C. (1970). *Self and ideal in a Guajiro life history* (Acta Ethnologicaet Linguistica No. 21, Series Americana No. 5). Vienna, Austria: Stiglmayr.

Watson, L. C., & Watson-Franke, M. (1985). *Interpreting life histories: An anthropological inquiry.* New Brunswick, NJ: Rutgers University Press.

Weinstein, D. (1979). *Bureaucratic opposition—Challenging abuses in the workplace.* New York, NY: Pergamon Press.

West-Sands, L. (1990). *Embracing the ugly child within: Life history of an incest survivor.* (Unpublished doctoral dissertation). Birmingham, AL: University of Alabama.

APPENDIX: SEMI-STRUCTURED INTERVIEW GUIDE

The following questions serve as a general framework for eliciting data about the key informant's life, cultural background, and the events surrounding the disclosure of incest.

The first set of questions is general in nature to put the person at ease. As the person becomes more comfortable and rapport is established, the questions become more focused on the sequences of communication in disclosure. (It is important to note that the interviewer does not need to ask questions about the nature of the sexual trauma because the focus of the study is on communication patterns of disclosure.)

The first set of questions is adapted from the interview guide used by West-Sands (1990).

The second set of questions dealing with disclosure was developed by the investigator for the purpose of this study.

1. Tell me about yourself, starting wherever you like (childhood, school-age, adolescence, adulthood).
   (The interview then progresses, eventually covering the informant's whole life.)
2. Tell me about the neighborhoods in which you lived while you were growing up. How would you describe the culture in the area where you grew up (ethnicity, norms, standards, cultural rules, educational level, income level)?
3. What does the future look like to you?
4. When you first began to sense that there was a problem, how did you account for it?
   Did you think anyone else in the family was aware?
   In what ways did your family members communicate with each other?
   What did you think would happen if you took no action?
5. What happened that you decided to tell someone about the incest?
   Whom did you tell and how did you decide to tell that person?
   What was that person's relationship to you?
6. What exactly did you say, and what was the person's response?
7. Paint the picture for me of where and when this conversation took place (the setting, who was present, was it planned or spontaneous).
8. What was it like to disclose (thoughts, feelings, expectations met/not met)?
   What do you most remember about that person's response to you?
9. How did your life change after disclosing?

CHAPTER SIX

THE STORIES OF US: USING LIFE HISTORIES TO INFORM PRACTICE

Adelita Cantu

MY STORY

Growing up in San Antonio, Texas, as a child, teenager, and young adult, I always remember myself as being obese. And because of that, many of the decisions that informed my behaviors were made in the context of my weight. Trying to get a doctor's excuse so I would not have to participate in physical education (PE) class, knowing that they were weighing all the children at school and making myself sick so I would not have to go to school that day, and as I got older, not wanting to go shopping with my friends as I did not want them to see what sizes I looked through.

I began to lose weight when I moved away from home. I have successfully kept off 100 pounds for over 30 years. However, I have found that my weight still informs decisions I make about clothes, about food, and about physical activity. Only this time it is because of a fear of gaining weight. Knowing what had happened in my life that led me to sustain a weight loss when I entered my doctoral studies and was contemplating my research interest, it quite naturally fell to wanting to better understand the intraperson mechanisms that contribute to the initiation and sustainability of a weight loss, particularly through engagement in physical activity.

WHY OLDER MEXICAN AMERICAN WOMEN?

As I entered my doctoral program, I expressed my research interest to my faculty advisor, and she was thrilled with my interest, principally because in San Antonio, Texas, where we lived, the type 2 diabetes prevalence rate is double the national average. The rate in San Antonio stands at 14%, double the national average of 7%, and it is the fourth leading cause of death in Bexar County, its largest city being San Antonio. Texas Hispanics of 65 years of age and older have a diabetes prevalence rate twice that of Whites and non-Hispanics—34.8% versus 17.0% (http://www.diabetes.org /in-my-community/local-offices/san-antonio-texas). Although the rates of Hispanic men and women do not differ significantly, I chose Hispanic women as my study group because as a Hispanic woman myself, my journey of discovery of the intraperson mechanisms that initiate and sustain weight loss through physical activity became more relatable and thus easier to put in context. In San Antonio, the Hispanic population is well over 90% of Mexican American descent. Again, my being a Hispanic woman of Mexican descent would ease the stress that may occur from being a "stranger in a strange land."

CHOOSING THE RESARCH QUESTION

Now that I had decided what I wanted to study, the next issue was what question I would ask to get me to answer my wonderment about intraperson mediators older Mexican American women used to initiate and sustain physical activity behavior. My faculty advisor told me to comb through the literature on this issue and make notes about what is known and what is not known. I spent many months reviewing literature relative to (a) importance of physical activity and health; (b) recommended dosage of physical activity throughout the life span; (c) frequency of physical activity across gender, ages, and race/ethnicity; and (d) facilitators and barriers to the initiation and maintenance of physical activity.

Lack of physical activity among Mexican American women of any age group is higher than the lack of physical activity observed among non-Hispanic Whites ages 70 to 79 (Kington & Smith, 1997). Crespo, Smit, Carter-Pokras, and Andersen (2001) reported that among older Mexican American women, the lack of leisure-time physical activity was lower than that reported for the general population. In addition, older Mexican American women show a marked decline in leisure-time activity after the age of 60 (Sundquist, Winkleby, & Pudaric, 2001). These facts confirmed that the lack of physical activity is high in older Mexican American women; however, it is even higher in older Mexican American women who are (a) of low socioeconomic status, (b) of a low educational level, and (c) less acculturated. This search of the literature assisted me to better define my population of interest: low-income, older Mexican American women who are currently physically inactive.

Specifically relative to the above facts about this population, I found numerous research articles that did describe facilitators and barriers relative to initiation and maintenance of physical activity in low-income Mexican American women who have low educational levels. For instance, Juarbe, Turok, and Pérez-Stable (2002) reported that perceived facilitators of physical activity for older Mexican American women included (a) improved health, (b) mental health, (c) family roles, (d) physical fitness/performance, and (e) easy access and transportation. Melillo and colleagues (2001) reported that motivation and social support were important facilitators.

Barriers included (a) time constraints from multiple roles; (b) personal health; (c) internal factors such as lack of motivation and fatigue; and (d) external factors such as transportation, weather, and cost (Juarbe, Turok, & Pérez-Stable, 2002). Older Mexican American women cited disability and health conditions, particularly arthritis and the fear of having a heart attack, as major barriers to sustained physical activity (Eyler et al., 1999; Gonzalez & Jirovec, 2001; Gonzales & Keller, 2004).

Knowing that the recognition and acknowledgment of facilitators and barriers to physical activity for a group of interest is important for designing interventions, I was perplexed at the physical activity intervention literature that I reviewed next. For instance, based on the literature that identified social support as a facilitator to physical activity, Keller and Gonzales (2001) and Poston and colleagues (2001) designed interventions for older Mexican American women that included a social support network. However, even when high levels of social support were designed as part of an investigation, significant attrition occurred. Similarly, Poston and colleagues, in an attempt to minimize attrition, assigned participants to a pre-established, ongoing social support network from work settings or neighborhoods. Despite this, investigators reported that, at the 6-month assessment, the attrition rate was similar for the treatment and control participants and that, at the 12-month assessment, the attrition rate in the treatment group was nearly twice that of the control group—47% and 28%, respectively. In addition, Poston and colleagues found that treated participants were not more active than the controls at 6 or 12 months.

I discussed my perplexity with my faculty advisor. From the literature, it seemed difficult to determine the extent to which decreasing perceived barriers related to encouraging the initiation and maintenance of physical activity behavior. It seems that previous interventions were tailored more in regard to delivery (social support) than in terms of content (the meaning of social support for the sample). Thus I arrived at the gap in the literature that would inform my research question, that being how correlates (facilitators and barriers) are conceptualized by the population of interest.

With this in mind, I went back to the literature. Kriska and Rexroad (1998) stated that for many minorities, taking time out of one's daily routine to focus on oneself, temporarily taking a break from one's obligations to family and work to exercise is less acceptable social behavior than in the majority mainstream culture. Eyler and colleagues (1998) reported that older Asian American, Native American, and Hispanic women believed that women of their ethnicity were "by nature" physically active due to their prescribed gender roles. Older Mexican American and Native American women have expressed similar sentiments (Gonzalez & Jirovec, 2001; Kriska & Rexroad, 1998). African American women appear more accepting of larger body sizes, and this acceptance may decrease motivation for physical activity (Carter-Nolan, Adams-Campbell, & Williams, 1996; Flynn & Fitzgibbon, 1998). Immigrant Mexican American women stated that being overweight symbolizes health or wealth (Juarbe, 1998). The literature reported more cultural beliefs that seemingly appeared to be barriers to physical activity. These findings told me that there appeared to be a host of sociocultural factors that play a role in how minority women conceptualize beliefs, which in turn inform their behavior relative to physical activity. Thus, a more robust understanding of the sociocultural meaning of constructs such as caregiving and social support and how they are interwoven with social and personal characteristics and life contexts was needed.

So my question became "What is the sociocultural context of physical activity in low-income, older Mexican American women?" Now that I have arrived at my question, my attention turned to how I would design my research to answer the question.

CHOOSING A METHODOLOGY

As I knew that I wanted to study culture, I wanted to get a content expert on my dissertation committee. I turned to a local liberal arts university and was pleased that a medical anthropologist agreed to be part of my committee. In discussions with her and by immersing myself in the literature on culture, I immediately realized that there is not a single definition of culture. But I focused on two things that were common in all definitions: (a) Culture is learned through interactions between the individual and his or her social networks, and (b) culture is integrative and functional, that is, it provides a sense of identity and framework that an individual uses to view, understand, and behave and passes on to succeeding generations. A key challenge that I had to keep in mind when choosing a methodology is that, as the definitions imply, culture is an abstraction in an individual's mind; people are usually not aware of the impact that their culture has on their thinking and behavior. Thus, I would face several challenges in the measurement of culture.

A common practice is to identify a proxy for culture (Kao, Hsu, & Clark, 2004). Race, ethnicity, language, nationality, and geographic location are most commonly selected as proxies for culture because of their convenient use and commonly assumed function as indicators of cultural beliefs and practices (Ahdieh & Hahn, 1996). However, culture is a very broad construct, too broad to use one variable as descriptive of an individual's culture. One thing that I reviewed in the literature is that researchers can examine and operationalize the numerous influences that vary by cultural groups. Yet, because these influences only have meaning within the context in which the person is living, it is important to integrate them back into the context from which they were extracted (Kao et al., 2004). As I had identified the gap in the literature to be the question of how correlates (facilitators and barriers of physical activity) are conceptualized by low-income, older Mexican American women, I decided a qualitative ethnographic formative work would provide a more robust understanding of how the cultural understanding of these correlates impacted the women's physical activity behavior. This would allow cultural beliefs to emerge from the data, rather than having such beliefs predetermined, as would happen in a quantitative study solely using one of the cultural proxies.

Rapid Assessment Process

When considering research designs, I was challenged with one big issue, time. As a result of various issues that included work and living location, I had to complete my data collection and analysis in a 3-month period. The anthropologist on my committee suggested a research design using the rapid assessment process (RAP). The RAP is an intensive, team-based, ethnographic inquiry using triangulation, iterative data analyses, and additional data collection to develop quickly a preliminary understanding of a situation from the insider's perspective. This allows a sufficient understanding of the situation to make preliminary decisions for the design and implementation of applied activities or additional research (Utarini, Winkvist, & Pelto, 2001).

Creswell (1998) identified compelling reasons for undertaking a qualitative study, and these reasons help to identify situations in which RAP is appropriate: (a) a topic needs to be explored, (b) the research question begins with "what," (c) there is a need for a detailed view, (d) there is a need to study individuals in their natural setting, and (e) there is a need to emphasize the researcher's role as a partner instead of an expert (Utarini et al., 2001).

The RAP research design was intended to yield descriptions of general sociocultural patterns of physical activity in inactive low-income, older Mexican American women. To use this design successfully, I knew that identifying key informants was a primary strategy to ensure that intracultural variation was limited (Utarini et al., 2001). This strategy was applied by (a) using a relatively narrow focus on a specific health problem (low levels of physical activity in low-income, older Mexican American women); (b) small samples of key informants and other respondents (40 older Mexican American women; 9 of the 40 as well as a geriatric primary care physician whose patient load included low-income, older Mexican American women were interviewed as case studies using life history); (c) a short period of field research (3 months); (d) interview guides that directed research; and (e) multiple methods of data collection (Utarini et al., 2001).

Location, Location, Location

I knew that I had to choose a sample from a location with the variables that I wanted to study and that would also ensure that intracultural variation would be limited. For this, I relied on my community roots, knowing the community that I was raised in and had worked in as a community health nurse for a number of years. I chose a senior center that I had worked with and is in a part of San Antonio that is low income and has some of the highest rates of cardiovascular disease and type 2 diabetes. The census tracts surrounding the senior center are home to approximately 30,972 individuals, of which 5,035 (16%) are over the age of 60. There are significantly more female older residents (60%) than male (40%). Mexican Americans are the predominant ethnic group (97%). One in three adults does not have either a high school diploma or a GED, with 1 in 12 adults not going beyond the eighth grade. One third (34%) of the residents fall below the federal poverty level, and this condition has remained unchanged during the past three decades (Good Samaritan Center, 2005). From the characteristics of the neighborhood and evidence from the literature, I selected this area as it suggested that the rates of physical inactivity among the neighborhood and the participants are high, impacting their health outcomes.

Why Life History Is Important

The anthropologist on my committee suggested that to truly understand the sociocultural context of physical activity within the daily lives of individuals, life history interviews would be instrumental to our research design. I began reading the literature on life histories and found that I wholeheartedly agreed with this method. The method made so much sense to me because I knew that, to really understand my almost obsessive behavior regarding my need to exercise and be physically active, you would have to know about my obesity as a youth and the importance of my sustained weight loss. Thus, to truly be embedded in your research, I found that having a robust understanding of your research design relative to your variables is critical for a true understanding of your findings.

Specifically, this method was chosen for the following reasons: (a) Sociocultural influences that are embedded in an individual's culture comprise a very broad construct, too broad for one variable to be descriptive of an individual's culture; (b) sociocultural influences that give cultural meaning to the individual only have meaning within that individual's context; and (c) life histories allow researchers to understand how individuals have interacted actively with the sociocultural influences in their context to structure their decisions about behaviors, particularly health behavior (Kao et al., 2004). Thus, I knew that I would obtain, using life history, some insight into the sociocultural influences that have informed my sample's decisions relative to physical activity.

Further, it is helpful to know that the field of anthropology has used life histories for many years and has found that it enables researchers to understand the interface between an individual's life and a specific sociocultural framework. Thus, life experiences can be linked to subsequent actions and behaviors (Gramling & Carr, 2004). Such meaning-centered, contextually based data provide insights applicable to the design of socially and culturally relevant intervention strategies and materials (Krumeich, Weijts, Reddy, & Meijer-Weitz, 2001).

For a sampling of how life histories have been used to design interventions, see Goldman and colleagues (2003), who used the life history methodology to plan context-rich, nonstereotyping intervention strategies and educational materials for a multicultural, working-class sample. Qualitative data that emerged relative to physical activity revealed that physical activity that appeared to lack a specific, tangible purpose was perceived as unnecessary (Goldman et al., 2003). The researchers then converted this finding into an operational guideline to teach the concept of incorporating sustained, intentional, and moderate physical activity that conferred health benefits in their daily lives.

Another way to realize interventions from this anthropological, life history approach is through the dialogue method (Krumeich et al., 2001). This method proposes interventions in which the target population is asked to react to the researcher's cultural analysis. This approach allows the target population (a) to assess whether the analysis parallels their own experiences; (b) to resist, correct, or refine the interpretation of their lives; and (c) to open up a discussion about the researcher's assumptions and norms (Krumeich et al., 2001). Two examples included efforts in Dominica to encourage mothers to breastfeed. After extensive fieldwork and discussion with the population by researchers, Dominican women suggested emphasizing cultural notions of motherhood (i.e., women as responsible mothers) for the promotion of breastfeeding among young women. In this way, gender relationships (men buying milk to show the community they take care of their children) could remain unchallenged while promoting breastfeeding in a culturally accepted way (Krumeich, 1994).

Fieldwork by Meyer-Weitz, Reddy, Weijts, van den Borne, and Kok (1998) showed that in selected South African communities, gender relationships interfere with compliance regarding condom use. Men's inclination to have multiple partners, their preference for penetration during sex, and their reluctance to use condoms as it is seen as wasting sperm put the men themselves and others at risk for sexually transmitted diseases (STDs) and HIV. For women, suggesting condom use is at odds with cultural norms of submissiveness and obedience toward men (Meyer-Weitz et al., 1998). After a dialogue with the community on the findings of their fieldwork, it was suggested that women point out to men that their clan would be served best by producing healthy offspring and that this was at odds with STD and HIV infections. Thus, a healthy offspring could compensate for the waste of sperm associated with condom use (Meyer-Weitz et al., 1998).

Ready to Get Started!

As I had worked with the chosen senior center previously, I felt very comfortable recruiting participants and specially establishing rapport with the participants that had consented to be interviewed. I began the interviews by gently asking and conversing with the participant about what she considered the highlights of her life. The answers varied in length of time; I never hurried the participant, just listening and offering prompts when I wished clarification or additional information on a highlight. Having heard some of their life histories before as a result of my previous work there allowed me to incorporate aspects of their lives into the prompts for additional information. This made the prompts clearer, more personal, and thus more understandable to the participant (Fleuriet, personal communication, July 16, 2004).

I then asked about how the participant defined physical activity. I made this transition clear in terms of how she believed that her life story had shaped the way she experiences physical activity. For example, one participant told me that when she was growing up with all brothers, she would run races with them and play baseball. As a transition, I asked her, knowing how she ran and played baseball as a youth, to give me her thoughts about physical activity now. This established the value of the participants' life stories in the context of this research.

The interviews were conducted in English as determined by the participant. The interviews were audio recorded and transcribed verbatim. I used text from the interviews to collect data regarding physical activity and cultural context. In addition to the interview, cultural inferences were generated through behavior and artifacts, the latter defined as the things that participants used when being physically active or inactive. To document interactions with participants, I relied on field notes that included transcripts of interviews and a journal of data-coding memos and observations of participants made during the interviews.

FINDINGS: THE EXCITING PART

The narratives of the participants' sociocultural context of physical activity provided details on organizing domains that included affinity for family and kinship relationships through close physical proximity and the embeddedness of gender roles (Cantu & Fleuriet, 2008). Family and kinship relationships are described as the primary unit within the participants' sociocultural context. This is not surprising and is descriptive of the traditional Mexican American family. The traditional Mexican American female gender role is to produce and take care of the family. What was surprising to me is that the embeddedness of this gender role was described as a process whereby common patterns or events that occurred during the participants' childhood seemed to have facilitated the "taking on" of the traditional female role.

In addition, active and dutiful caregiving was overarching throughout the organizing domains (Cantu & Fleuriet, 2008). Active and dutiful caregiving seemed to be a substantive part of the development of the affinity for family and kinship relationships and gender roles. Based on the narratives, I have defined *active caregiving* as assistance with activities of daily living while *dutiful caregiving* is described as "the being there aspect of caring," or as being physically available and present to family members, even though providing active caregiving is not necessary.

Affinity for Family and Kinship Relationships

The life history of each of the low-income, older Mexican American women had similar patterns that seemed to reinforce their development of affinity for family and kinship relationships. According to Spradley (1980), a taxonomic analysis showed that those relationships included (a) a childhood that was very happy; (b) a strict father; (c) an extreme emotional attachment to one or both parents, grandparents, and siblings; (d) a large immediate and extended family; (e) being reared in a low socioeconomic status household; and (f) marriage at an early age. For this sample of women, the mean number of siblings was seven and the mean age for marriage was 18.7 years. One woman stated,

> It was a two-bed room, one bathhouse and there were five children. My two brothers, their bedroom was the dining room with the two beds on each side. We had the biggest bedroom because we were three girls and one closet, so we shared that. We lived right next door to a grocery store, so the roaches would come all the time, it was a wooden house, it was just terrible. But we didn't care, we were having so much fun.

Another stated that although they lived in poverty, she was happy: "I was real happy, at home I had dinner, just to be around the house helping my mother with the things." Still another participant, Delia, stated, "We lived in a house and we were 12 . . . . I was very close to my mother, I was not very close to my father though, I was close to my mother, very close."

Family and kinship relationships were very much described by physical proximity; being there was a necessity, and the togetherness was important to being a family. All of the women in the sample lived within a three-mile radius of a family member, usually a daughter or parent. Five had made a geographical move from another state back to San Antonio to be closer to family, and only two who made that move did it because of the need to provide active caregiving for elderly parents.

One woman stated that as she was growing up in Wisconsin, her parents made a move back to Texas to care for their parents:

But then afterwards my mom decided to move back because of my grandma, the reason being that my grandma kept saying, "I'm getting older and you are not going to see me and you are too far away," so my mom decided to move back to be close to her parents.

This same woman, when later living in Chicago with her husband, made the same move: "Also you know, my parents were here, everybody in my family was here, so we moved back over here." When asked how her husband felt about this, Ana stated,

The reasons, I think he thought it was better, they have better paying jobs over there [in Chicago] and stuff that you can do better over there, but I guess it's really, sometimes it's not all about money, you know, it's about your family and how you feel and where you want to be, so this is where I wanted to be.

As an exemplar of the abstractness of culture, one woman stated that she had moved closer to her parents but could not articulate a reason, other than that she liked the location. "Well, I loved to be here near my parents, but that's not the reason. We moved back because, I don't know . . . . We just moved, I don't know why, you know."

Embeddedness of Gender Role Expectations

Even though I was a Mexican American and knew the cultural heritage, the life histories were enlightening for me and deepened my understanding of how the heritage continues. I know that the role of traditional Mexican American woman is to reproduce and take care of the family. Her job is to cook, clean, and care for the children. A good wife is submissive and takes orders from her husband. She is also tolerant of her husband's behavior. But I did not realize how much that role expectation is reinforced through parents and husbands.

One participant discussed how her father's strictness and adherence to gender roles affected her mother.

Because my mother had so much problems, because my dad wouldn't let her become an American citizen. She wanted to become an American citizen and he said no. She wanted to learn how to drive and he said no. She wanted to get a job to help out and he said no.

One reported being beaten by an older brother several times.

> Sometimes he would come home from work and say, "Don't you have anything else to make?" Because he probably didn't like what I had made, and sometimes I would make eggs for him and if I broke the yellow thing he would get so mad. He would get so mad and hit . . . I would talk to myself, I wouldn't tell him, "Well, if you don't like it you can make it yourself," but I wouldn't say it, you know. He was the one that had the authority. And then my mother had to, I don't know, I think sometimes my mother gives them too much authority.

Imelda also described how her father had an impact on her pursuit of a career.

> When I was single . . . I wanted to be an RN [registered nurse], but my father did not want me to. He didn't like it, said it was taking care of old men, I don't know what his thoughts were, but now that I took care of him through his elderly years, I told him, see, and you didn't want me to be an RN.

One participant stated that her husband allowed her to learn English on the condition that she use it only to better care for the children but not to go to work.

Interestingly, an outlier to having expectations reinforced by marriage, Carmen spoke of how her father's patriarchal authority led to her expectations for her relationship with her ex-husband. Because he was Anglo, she described how difficult it was for her to overcome that expectation.

> In 1968 I met my future husband on a blind date. So I thought, well, he's going to take care of me like my dad takes care of me, he's going to buy my underwear, buy my pants, buy my bras, turn on the electricity; well, it was a rude awakening for me, because he was from San Francisco, and we got married here in San Antonio and then we moved to San Francisco. So when we got our first apartment he said, "You need to call the gas company." And I said, "Why?" He said, "Because we need gas in the apartment." "Well, can't you do it? Dad always did it, what do you mean I have to do it?" It was terrible. I hated him for that. Because he made me do things that I was just not used to.

Active and Dutiful Caregiving Issues

This was the most interesting aspect of the life history narratives. Although it is well documented in the literature that caregiving is a barrier to the initiation and maintenance of physical activity, it was not until I fully analyzed the participants' life history stories relative to how caregiving is embedded into their lives did I fully understand how they conceptualized caregiving.

One woman, who is primary caregiver to three of her grandchildren, when asked whether she felt the needs of her family and grandchildren were a burden to her, stated, "It's my responsibility . . . . That is something that I want to teach my kids . . . if they see that their brother needs something, if he is sick or needs food, then they need to be there for him." When asked who taught her that it was her responsibility, she stated that is was her grandmother, who had 12 children.

Imelda spoke of her caregiving to both her aging parents with pride: "I took real good care of him, both of them for as long as I did, I am glad I had that special time with them."

An exemplar of the perception of the role of caregiving in their lives, one participant who cares for a disabled husband and is the primary caregiver of an adopted granddaughter with a history of severe asthma, also works part time from 6:00 a.m. to 9:00 a.m. as a housekeeper and then babysits for three of her other grandchildren after returning home from work. When asked how that came about, she stated that at first, the kids took turns going to each grandmother's house. However, she stated that she would babysit all the time because the other grandmother "works more than I do. I only work in the mornings, so I can do it full-time." Further, she said that she told the parents of the children (the father is her son), "I will take care of the kids because I know you guys need to go have your jobs, and you have to go home and take care of the kids, and you need your time too." The participant did not seem to consider her job and then coming home to take care of three children at the same level of hardship as it would be for her son and daughter-in-law.

In an excellent example of dutiful caregiving and one that I was able to link from the participant's life history to thoughts on physical activity, this participant, who had been married twice with a 15-year break between marriages, explained why, after going to the gym for 15 years and exercising, she has stopped since her second marriage.

Participant: It's not that he keeps me from going; maybe it's because of my culture, I feel like I have to be waiting on him or being with him and not doing my own thing, I don't know.

PI: And has your husband ever said, say if you ever wanted to go to the gym, I'm going to the gym, would he stop you . . .

Gloria: I don't know, because I have never given him that opportunity.

When asked how she came to this belief, the participant stated that she learned this from her mother: "She was always very good with her husband, and she is always telling me to be good to him, to be careful, serve him, blah, blah, blah . . . . She comes to visit and she tells me the same thing."

In another example, another participant described getting an emergency telephone call from Houston that her uncle was gravely ill. Notice how many times the word *there* occurs.

> I told my husband, "Let's go over there," so we threw some clothes together and took off to Houston and got over there to the hospital and still got to talk to my uncle, and he knew I was there and I called my mom. We got over there and I told my mom that he was very serious and, "You need to get over here." So the whole family went over there, my aunt, my brother, my mom, my cousins, everybody went over there, and I think we were over there about a week. Everybody went over there and they were sleeping there in the chairs waiting, and when he passed away we were all there with him.

Issues With Findings

I was excited about the findings of this life history study because it provided me with a starting point for understanding how older Mexican American women perceived physical activity within their sociocultural context, centered on how family and kinship relationships, gender role expectations, and active and dutiful caregiving influenced behavior such as physical activity. This study demonstrated the value of using the life history methodology for exploring the sociocultural context of an individual. It certainly has increased my understanding of how individuals actively interact with those sociocultural influences to structure their decisions about behaviors, particularly physical activity. This understanding is vital to the design of successful, culturally relevant interventions that can work to decrease health disparities.

For instance, previously cited interventions for older Mexican American women have had limited success, possibly due to the researchers' understanding of family issues and caregiving as a barrier being based on the notion that the pursuit of physical activity takes time away from caring for the family, thus suggesting providing daycare as an intervention. However, if physical activity is understood as a pursuit that keeps women physically and emotionally away from their families, not "*being present*" for their families, the problem is not surmounted by daycare.

This finding prompted my next research study, also using life history methodology, about the impact that "being with aspect of caring" has on the maintenance of older Mexican American women who are physically active. Expanding the qualitative work would examine the sociocultural influences that they use to maintain their behavior relative to physical activity, particularly relative to whether "being with aspect of caring" remains a cultural theme and, if so, how these women maintain physical activity as a life choice. In particular, how do they problem-solve the issue of being there relative to continuing physical activity? Additionally, if the theme of "being with" is absent among women who are physically active, additional questions will need to be addressed in order to develop appropriate screening tools. Such screening tools could help to identify women whose decisional frame is highly influenced by "being with" versus those whose decisional frame is influenced by something else. These screening tools would assist in the development of interventions that are tailored to fit Mexican American women's decisional frame.

Limitation Issues

It is important to keep in mind that, as with any qualitative work, the perceptions reported by verbal statements made by individuals are subject to fabrication, exaggeration, distortion, and predisposition to agreement with researcher. In addition, at times what people say and what they actually do differ.

Finally, the intricacies of culture, the sociocultural influences on culture, and how they interface with an individual's behavior, particularly physical activity behavior, are uniquely constructed by the individual. In addition, that construction of behavior is fluid and flexible, depending on real-time contextual influences. Thus, although the present findings were very encouraging relative to the insights into the sociocultural context of older Mexican American women and how it impacts physical activity behavior, use of the findings must be considered in the context in which they were derived.

SUMMARY

The conceptual orientation of this study was based on the idea that women of a specific racial or ethnic background have perceptions, attitudes, and values about physical activity that are unique to their culture. Although culture is very complex, using the life history methodology elicited themes that included affinity for family and kinship relationships through close physical proximity and embedded gender roles, describing the sociocultural context of physical activity in this sample of older Mexican American women. The traditional Mexican American female gender role is to take care of the family. This gender role was embedded as a common pattern during childhood and facilitated the traditional female role in this sample of women.

In addition, the theme of active and dutiful caregiving was prominent throughout all of the interviews and had its roots in both the development of the affinity for family and kinship relationships and the embeddedness of gender roles. Dutiful caregiving is described as being physically available to a family member, although active caregiving is not required. Interestingly enough, when I presented this study, particularly the finding of dutiful caregiving, at a nursing conference, one attendee told me that she had finally gotten information that was useful to her practice. She told me that she had seen the concept of dutiful caregiving in her practice but had not been able to name it until now; naming it assisted her to better communicate with her patients and their perceived barriers to care. This, more than anything else, confirmed for me the value of life histories.

REFERENCES

Ahdieh, L., & Hahn, R. A. (1996). Use of terms race, ethnicity, and national origin: A review of articles in the *American Journal of Public Health, 1980–1989. Ethnicity and Health, 1*, 95–98.

Cantu, A. G., & Fleuriet, K. J. (2008). Sociocultural context of physical activity in older Mexican American women. *Hispanic Health Care International, 6*, 1–20.

Carter-Nolan, P. L., Adams-Campbell, L. L., & Williams, J. (1996). Recruitment strategies for Black women at risk for non-insulin-dependent diabetes mellitus into exercise protocols: A qualitative assessment. *Journal of the National Medical Association, 88*, 558–562.

Crespo, C. J., Smit, E., Carter-Pokras, O., & Andersen, R. (2001). Acculturation and leisure-time inactivity in Mexican American adults: Results from NHANES III, 1988–1984. *American Journal of Public Health, 91*, 1254–1257.

Creswell, J. (1998). *Qualitative inquiry and research design: Choosing among five traditions.* Thousand Oaks, CA: Sage.

Eyler, A. A., Baker, E., Cromer, L., King, A. C., Brownson, R. C., & Donatelle, R. J. (1998). Physical activity and minority women: A qualitative study. *Health Education and Behavior, 25*, 640–652.

Eyler, A., Brownson, R., Donatelle, R., King, A., Brown, D., & Sallis, J. (1999). Physical activity social support in middle and older aged minority women: Results from a U.S. survey. *Social Science and Medicine, 49*, 781–789.

Flynn, K. J., & Fitzgibbon, M. (1998). Body images and obesity risk among Black females: A review of the literature. *Behavioral Medicine, 20,* 13–24.

Goldman, R., Hunt, M. K., Allen, J. D., Hauser, S., Emmons, K., Maeda, M., & Sorensen, G. (2003). The life history interview method: Applications to intervention development. *Health Education and Behavior, 30,* 564–581.

Gonzales, A., & Keller, C. S. (2004). *Mi familia viene primero* (My family comes first): Physical activity issues in older Mexican American women. *Southern Online Journal of Nursing, 5*(4), 1–21.

Gonzalez, B. C., & Jirovec, M. M. (2001). Elderly Mexican women's perceptions of exercise and conflicting role responsibility. *International Journal of Nursing Studies, 38,* 45–49.

Good Samaritan Center. (2005). *Programs: Senior and adult services.* San Antonio, TX: Author. Retrieved from http://www.goodsamcenter.org

Gramling, L. F., & Carr, R. L. (2004). Lifelines: A life history methodology. *Nursing Research, 53*(3), 207–210.

Juarbe, T. (1998). Cardiovascular disease-related diet and exercise experiences of immigrant Mexican women. *Western Journal of Nursing Research, 20,* 765–782.

Juarbe, T., Turok, X. P., & Pérez-Stable, E. J. (2002). Perceived benefits and barriers to physical activity among older Latina women. *Western Journal of Nursing Research, 24,* 868–886.

Kao, H. S., Hsu, M., & Clark, L. (2004). Conceptualizing and critiquing culture in health research. *Journal of Transcultural Nursing, 15,* 269–277.

Keller, C. S., & Gonzales, A. (2001, October). Effects of two frequencies of walking on cardiovascular risk factor reduction in Mexican American women. *Research in Nursing and Health, 24*(5), 390–401.

Kington, R. S., & Smith, J. P. (1997). Socioeconomic status and racial and ethnic differences in functional status associated with chronic diseases. *American Journal of Public Health, 87,* 805–810.

Kriska, A., & Rexroad, A. (1998). The role of physical activity in minority populations. *Women's Health Issues, 8,* 98–103.

Krumeich, A. (1994). *The blessings of motherhood. Health, pregnancy, and child care in Dominica.* Amsterdam: Het Spinhuis.

Krumeich, A., Weijts, W., Reddy, P., & Meijer-Weitz, A. (2001). The benefits of anthropological approaches for health promotion research and practice. *Health Education Research, 16,* 121–130.

Melillo, K. D., Williamson, E., Houde, S. C., Futrell, M., Read, C. Y., & Campasano, M. (2001). Perceptions of older Latino adults regarding physical fitness, physical activity, and exercise. *Journal of Gerontological Nursing, 27,* 38–46.

Meyer-Weitz, A., Reddy P., Weijts, W., van den Borne, B., & Kok, G. (1998). Sociocultural contexts of sexually transmitted diseases in South Africa: Implications for health education programmes. *AIDS Care, 10*(Suppl 1), S39–S55.

Poston, W. S. C., Haddock, K., Olvera, N. E., Suminski, R. R., Reeves, R. S., Dunn, J. K., & Foreyt, J. P. (2001). Evaluation of a culturally appropriate intervention to increase physical activity. *American Journal of Health Behavior, 25,* 396–406.

Spradley, J. P. (1980). *Participant observation.* New York, NY: Holt, Rinehart & Winston.

Sundquist, J., Winkleby, M. A., & Pudaric, S. (2001). Cardiovascular disease risk factors among older Black, Mexican-American, and White women and men: An analysis of NHANES III, 1988–1994. *Journal of the American Geriatrics Society, 49,* 109–116.

Utarini, A., Winkvist, A., & Pelto, G. H. (2001, Winter). Appraising studies in health using rapid assessment procedures (RAP): Eleven critical criteria. *Human Organization, 60*(4), 390–400.

CHAPTER SEVEN

THEORIZED LIFE HISTORIES: MASCULINITY AND MALE SUICIDE

Jo River and Murray J. Fisher

*T*his chapter reports on an empirical study of two men who engaged in nonfatal suicide. It is part of a larger study of 18 Australian men. These initial cases were used s to assess the suitability of life history method, together with a theoretical framework of gender relations, for understanding the relationship between masculinity and male suicide. The broad objective of the research program is to inform suicide prevention programs and health interventions.

The life history method can provide rich documentation of an individual's life and is a recognized method for examining issues of gender. It makes visible the wider influence of social, cultural, and historical factors (Miller, 2000; Plummer, 2001). Gender relations theory has emerged from the field of sociology and is able to capture the complex nature of gender within a life story. The two are woven together into the theorized life history, which can illuminate the dynamic interplay of personal agency and social structure in the making of masculinity. This method has demonstrated value in research on men and masculinity (Plummer, 2001).

The two theorized life histories reported here reveal that masculinity was a mechanism that mediated between suicidal behavior and other social factors such as employment status and marital breakdown.

WHY EXAMINE THE GENDERED NATURE OF MALE SUICIDE?

National and international statistics reveal a striking gender difference in suicide rates worldwide. Male suicide deaths exceed female deaths in every country except China (WHO, 2011). This is particularly remarkable given the wide geographical, cultural, religious, and other social variations between countries. The gender difference in suicide rates within Australia mirrors global patterns, with male suicide fatalities exceeding female suicide fatalities across regional, ethnic, and socioeconomic groups (Page, Morrell, Taylor, Dudley, & Carter, 2007; Tatz, 2005; Taylor, Page, Morrell, Harrison, & Carter, 2005a, 2005b).

The Lay of the Land

Prior to gathering data, I wanted to gain an overview of the suicide research. I particularly wanted to understand the extent to which it gave a satisfactory account of the observed sex difference in suicide. In brief, there is a substantial body of literature on suicide that can be broadly synthesized into the two opposing discourses of medicine and social science, with the psychiatric discourse representing an alternate medical dialogue that mediates between biological dysfunction and suicidal behavior. Biomedical research has largely focused on the search for innate biological distinctions between men and women. Sophisticated studies have primarily examined the relationship between suicide and serotonin levels, serotonin genes, and testosterone. The link between these biological markers and elevated rates of male suicide remains uncertain. In the psychiatric literature, suicide is viewed as an observable symptom of depression (Psychiatry Online, 2008). The observed higher rates of male suicide across all diagnostic groups have led to the category "male" becoming a designated risk factor for suicide in the biopsychosocial model of suicide (Mann, 2002). There is little explanation of why being male is so risky. The social research literature finds higher rates of male suicide fatalities associated with social factors such as employment status, relationship breakdown, sexuality, and suicide method (Smalley, Scourfiled, & Greenland, 2005). What is not clear is how this relates to gender.

In spite of the conspicuous sex difference in suicide rates, the issue of gender has rarely been examined within the social research literature. An Irish study by Anne Cleary (2005) presents the most comprehensive analyses. Cleary (2005) interviewed men who had engaged in nonfatal suicide and presents convincing evidence that hegemonic masculine ideals, which depict disclosure as weak and unmasculine, constrain emotional expression and prevent help seeking in suicidal men. Cleary (2005) made only brief links between male suicide and social institutions such as family and the workplace. These may be "key" factors in understanding the social process of constructing masculinity (Messerschmidt, 2000).

There is growing recognition that the social construction of masculinity is a major factor in men's physical and mental health outcomes; nevertheless, the gendered nature of suicide has long been ignored in social research and health service planning.

CHOOSING A METHOD

Exploring the relationship between male suicidal behavior and the social process of constructing masculinity led to distinct theoretical, methodological, and ethical considerations. To examine masculinity, I needed a clear definition of gender. I also needed a qualitative method that could investigate individual men's experiences while making the social processes of constructing masculinity visible. Finally, the sensitive nature of the research called for careful consideration of participant safety throughout the recruitment and interview process.

Defining Gender

Gender represents one of the most significant "organizing" principles of our social world; it structures individual identity, social interactions, and social institutions (Wharton, 2005). However, the concept of gender has been "fiercely contested" within the social sciences over the past century (Connell, 2005).

In the 1950s, sex role theory dominated sociological discourses of gender. Talcott Parsons, a key proponent of "sex-role theory," theorized that children were socialized into complementary and mutually exclusive male or female roles, based on sex at birth. Sex role theory set normative standards for men and women and suggested that social dysfunction occurred when an individual was unable to, or unwilling to, fulfill his or her assigned sex role (Carrigan, Connell, & Lee, 1985). The conservatism of sex role theory was challenged in the 1970s by prominent feminist thinkers (Carrigan et al., 1985). It was criticized for implying that men and women formed distinct but equal groups and for making invisible the unequal power relations between men and women (Carrigan et al., 1985; Connell, 2005). Feminist academics were instrumental in replacing concepts of sex roles with those of patriarchy. Gay scholars also critiqued the idea that men formed a homogenous group, pointing to the dominant ideology of compulsory heterosexuality that created distinctly unequal power relations amongst men (Carrigan et al., 1985).

By the mid-1980s, critiques of the sex role theory began to inform pro-feminist scholars concerned with issues of masculinity (Carrigan et al., 1985). The work of pro-feminist, feminist, and gay scholars was synthesized and integrated into a "systematic sociological theory of gender," which became known as gender relations theory (Connell & Messerschmidt, 2005). This theory was articulated by Connell (1987), in "Gender and Society" (Connell & Messerschmidt, 2005).

Gender relations theory described gender as the "structure of social relations" based on "reproductive distinctions between bodies" (Connell, 2002). Unlike sex role theory, it is able to give an account of the power relations between men and women as well as among men and among women (Connell & Messerchmidt, 2005). It also contends that multiple patterns of masculinity emerge from the interaction of gender with other major social structures of class, ethnicity, sexuality, and religion (Connell, 2002). Hegemonic masculinity describes the particular pattern of masculinity that is culturally idealized and honored; it is the "standard against which other forms of manhood are measured and evaluated" (Kimmel, 1994). Aligning with the dominant ideology of manhood secures for men the power to control and oppress women as well as subordinate other men who fail to conform to hegemonic standards (Ashe, 2007). Whereas existing social structures may restrain or facilitate achievement of hegemonic masculinity, men are themselves agents who actively engage in perpetuating or resisting existing "gendered social structures" and dominant ideologies of manhood (Messerschmidt, 2000).

Over the past 20 years, gender relations theory has become increasingly influential. It provides a vehicle for understanding patterns of difference, both among men as well as between men and women (Connell, & Messerschmidt, 2005; Schofield, Connell, Walker, Wood, & Butland, 2000). For the study of male suicidal behavior, gender relations theory presents a theoretical framework that has the potential to elucidate relations of power, subordination, resistance, and complicity among men, and between men and women, which may be significant in understanding the gendered nature of suicide.

Constructing Theorized Life Histories

I chose the life history method as a qualitative research method. Life histories are collected through in-depth interviews that allow respondents to "move back and forth" in their narrative and meaningfully organize, describe, and explain key life events and situations within the wider significance of their life stories (Miller, 2000; Plummer, 2001). Although it is a time-consuming method (Connell, 2010), it provides rich descriptions of an individual life and simultaneously allows insight into collective social processes (Connell, 2005; Messerschmidt, 1999). It can retain the whole individual story and locate it within the wider social, cultural, and historical moment (Connell, 2010; Plummer, 2001). The life history method is arguably an ideal method for understanding the lives of individual men who engage in suicidal behavior, the meaning of suicidal behavior within the context of their lives, and the relationship between male suicide and social processes such as gender.

Used together, gender relations theory and life history method provide a "powerful tool" for capturing the dynamic interplay of personal agency and social structure in the making of masculinity (Connell, 2000). Theorized life histories have demonstrated value in research on men and masculinity (Plummer, 2001). Notable studies include Donaldson and Poynting's (2007) *Ruling Class Men*, which presents a fascinating account of the lives of wealthy men; James Messerschmidt's (2000) *Nine Lives*, which illuminates issues related to violent crime in adolescent males, and Michael Messner's (1995) *Power at Play*, which provides a provocative appraisal of male athletes in professional sport. Theorized life histories have also been used to study the interplay of gender and health, for example, Gary Dowsett's (1996) *Practicing Desire*, which investigated sexual practice within the gay community of Nullangardie, Australia, in the era of AIDS; Fisher and Chilko's (2012) small study of the construction of masculinities in obese men; and Gallagher, Marshall, and Fisher's (2008, 2010) studies of women's recovery from an acute coronary syndrome.

Selecting Participants and Maintaining Safety

Some decisions regarding participant selection were fairly clear. They had to be Australian males who had survived a suicidal act. What constituted a suicidal act was more problematic. Not all men who engage in suicidal behavior come into contact with medical services (Elnour & Harrison, 2008). As such, the seriousness of their suicide attempt may not be ascertained. To add to the problem, medical professionals themselves regularly assume lower intent based on gender, suicide method, and a nonfatal outcome (Jaworski, 2007). Male suicide is often considered more serious and intentional than female suicide (Jaworski, 2007). The use of suicide methods that are less lethal, such as medication overdose, are commonly viewed as "cries for help," although these same methods contribute a major portion of suicide deaths and nonfatal suicide injuries (Jaworski, 2007). Canetto and Safinofsky (1998) note that suicide outcome is wrongly conflated with intent. Men and women who die by suicide may or may not have intended it. Similarly, those who engaged in nonfatal suicide may not have expected to live. Considering these issues, I decided to recruit men who identified their suicidal act as serious action to cause death, whether or not it was validated by a medical professional. I chose to exclude men who were currently suicidal. I hoped to avoid exacerbation of any current suicidal feelings.

Given that this area of research is undertheorized, exclusion criteria based on factors such as age might be irrelevant to the study of "masculinities" and male suicide. I chose only to exclude men under the age of 18 years or over the age of 80 years because youth or the frailties of aging could potentially accentuate the risk of harm to these participants. Although it was not desirable, non-English speaking men were also excluded. I only speak English, and my limited financial resources precluded the use of interpreters.

Men who have engaged in suicidal behavior often face discrimination in both the community and health care settings (Talseth, Lindseth, Jacobsson, & Norberg, 1999). I anticipated that men would be reluctant to come forward without reassurance. To provide such reassurance, a passive network sampling technique was chosen. This sampling technique allowed recruitment of participants via "word of mouth" through health professional colleagues. Colleagues were asked to discuss the research with friends and contacts who met the entry criteria. A "Participant Information Statement" sheet was sent out, and potential participants were invited to contact the researcher for further information. This recruitment method brought two men forward.

I later revised this recruitment strategy in the larger study of 18 men. Word of mouth recruitment was laborious and slow. I tried recruiting through organizations supporting suicidal men and women. I thought this would provide the reassurance and support necessary. This method still required constant networking and yielded few participants. Finally, I gained permission to place advertisements in local newspapers. Recruitment happened very quickly by this means. It had the added advantage of recruiting men who had no links with health services, which allowed me to investigate the reasons for men not seeking help.

Interviewing men who have previously been suicidal poses particular ethical concerns. Participant safety was paramount, and strategies to eliminate or minimize any negative impact had to be carefully considered and built into the study procedure. This issue became particularly important when I began recruiting through newspapers. To avoid recruiting men with current suicidal ideation and a protracted history of mental illness, I required participants to identify themselves as having recovered both physically and psychologically following engagement in nonfatal suicide.

I informed participants of the risks of being involved in the study. I also sent out a "Participant Information Statement," which frankly detailed the purpose of the study and study procedures and warned participants of the potential for distress when recounting life events. These issues were again reiterated verbally when I discussed the study with participants. It was made clear that consent was only provisional and participants were free to stop the interview at any time and withdraw consent without explanation or negative consequences. A referral pathway to a mental health nurse and doctor was prearranged for those participants who might require immediate support or debriefing. Both of these health professionals had considerable experience working with suicidal men.

Interviews were conducted at a time and private location chosen by the participant to maximize comfort. Many of these initial interviews were conducted in a quiet and private room at the university. Later, I also undertook interviews in men's houses. For these interviews, I followed strict guidelines to protect my safety. This included a log book detailing the name and address of the participant. I also contacted a fellow researcher before and after the interview. In all the interviews (18), only one man showed any distress. With his permission, I referred him to one of the prearranged health professionals.

Given the stigma associated with suicide and the personal nature of life history data, identification of participants in any publications or conferences was of particular concern. Participant anonymity was protected by the use of pseudonyms and through the editing of transcripts to remove any identifying data, such as names of friends or relatives and place names. In addition, I recruited participants from separate sources. They had no knowledge of, or connection to, one another. It is anticipated that only those in the study would recognize themselves in the data.

Carrying Out the Interviews

The interviews were semi-structured conversations. In the opening question, I did not directly refer to suicidal behavior. Considering the stigma associated with nonfatal suicidal behavior, I did not wish to immediately confront participants with this question. Given that participants were aware that they had come to discuss suicide, I chose to let them approach that part of their lives within the course of their own story. I simply asked participants to tell me about their lives from whichever point in time they wished and to highlight events that were important to them. I did not develop specific questions. Rather, I identified areas of interest to guide my questions. These areas concerned family relationships, school life, friendships, work history, personal relationships, life stressors leading to suicidal behavior, suicidal behavior, and subsequent recovery. If participants did not cover these issues in the telling of their life story, I would tentatively question them.

In the initial study, both men began with a chronological history of events leading up to their engagement in suicidal behavior and subsequent recovery. They covered the major points of their stories in the first half hour of the interview. Stories were then retold in more detail, moving forward and backward in time to emphasize the relationship between events. I asked questions to clarify points or seek more detail of a particular event. Interviews took between 1 and 3 hours.

A Woman Interviewing Men

Considering that the focus of this study is masculinity and male suicide, the issue of my own female gender is perhaps relevant. I was often asked by fellow researchers how being a woman and interviewing men impacted the interview process. I understand that researcher characteristics such as gender, age, class, and race can "shape" the interaction between researcher and participant (Plummer, 2001). Yet, as Plummer (2001, p. 156) observed, to "purge" the research process of all these factors is to rid it of "human life." It is impossible to take yourself out of the equation. A man could feel more comfortable talking to another man about sensitive issues such as suicide. However, going back to the theory of gender relations, it is important to recognize that men construct masculinity in relation to other men as well as to women (Ashe, 2007). Given that emotional expression and suicide survival are depicted as weak and unmasculine (Jaworski, 2007), a man who is vulnerable to being demoted within the masculine order might feel less threatened by a female interviewer. In either case, the gender of the researcher has some impact on the interview process. I can only say that the men recruited into this study appeared to be open, honest, and willing to speak freely on very personal and sensitive subjects. They did not appear to hold back on account of my gender.

ANALYZING THE INTERVIEW DATA

This section examines how to analyze life history narratives within a theoretical framework of gender relations. First, an individual's position in the gender order is complex and frequently inconsistent (Connell, 2002). Depending on the particular social practices within an institution, men and women may be alternately honored or subordinated (Connell, 2002). For instance, a man who experiences promotion and privilege at the workplace may be socially subordinated by homosexual practice in his private life (Messerschmidt, 2000). To capture the complex nature of gender within an individual narrative, Connell (2002) suggests that researchers examine gender relations within the four distinguishing substructures of power, production, symbolism, and emotional relations (Connell, 2005).

Using the Gender Substructures

I used Connell's four gender substructures to examine all of the life histories. This presented me with a practical and systematic approach for examining gender within life history accounts. I could look for descriptions with the narratives that related to power, production, cathexis (emotional relations), and symbolism. However, this structured analysis was undertaken with the understanding that the substructures of gender presented by Connell are not absolute or clear categories and that any analysis of gender must also "go beyond gender" (Connell, 2005) to illuminate the complexities of suicide and masculinity. This approach does not preclude a holistic understanding of the gendered story but seeks to capture the complex and contradictory nature of gender relations in the lives of each participant (Connell, 2002).

The four dimensions of gender are not discrete categories, but constantly fluctuating and overlapping subjective experiences within the gender system (Fisher, 2006). For example, the emotional and power relations between men cannot necessarily be separated in issues such as homophobic violence. Gender itself is not a discrete category. It "intersects" with other key social structures such as ethnicity, class, and religion (Connell 2005, p. 75). For example, a man may be subordinated or distinguished on the basis of color or social class (Connell, 2002).

Power Relations

Gendered power relations describe the "direct and indirect ways" in which men and women are controlled by others, for the benefit of others (Connell, 1987). Examining power relationships within life history narratives can illuminate the means by which institutional power and dominant discourses restrain or facilitate social action (Connell, 2002). It can also show how men and women variously comply with, resist, or contest such power (Connell, 2002). For example, it can demonstrate the way in which men use dominant ideologies, financial power, and even physical power to dominate women and how that domination is accepted, contested, resisted, or overcome (Connell, 2002).

Production or Work Relations

Production is an important structure in which gender is created, maintained, and negotiated (McDowell, 2003). There is a gender division of labor that depicts particular work as masculine and other work as feminine. This division of labor operates both within paid work, as well as between paid and unpaid labor (Connell, 2002). For example, construction work is typically depicted as masculine, whereas caring professions and unpaid domestic work are seen as more suitable for women. Scrutinizing life histories for work relations draws attention to how individuals negotiate the gendered social norms that surround work practices.

Cathexis or Emotional Relations

Cathexis is considered another key "dimension of gender." Analyzing the emotional relationships between men and women, as well as among men and among women can bring to light complex emotional ties, contradictions, and hostilities such as heterosexuality and misogyny, homo-social behavior and homophobia (Connell, 2002).

Symbolic Relations

Connell (2002) describes symbolism as the fourth dimension of gender. Studying symbolic relations in life histories draws attention to how gender discourses are symbolized through language, clothing, gestures, and the media. Consider, for example, the media depictions of war heroes and sporting stars that epitomize hegemonic masculinity (Connell, 2005), which in turn make combat trousers and sports shirts acceptable items of clothing for men. However, men who dress in drag do not necessarily occupy a socially feminized place in other gender substructures (Connell, 1998).

Applications

Other researchers in the field of men and masculinities have applied this structural analysis to understand the construction of masculinity within various populations and social institutions (Connell, 2005; Fisher, 2009; Fisher & Chilko, 2012; Messerschmidt, 2000; Schofield & Goodwin, 2006).

Collective Analysis

In theory building research, data saturation can occur once "theoretical saturation takes place," and new data do not generate new theory (Miller, 2000, p. 124). It was not anticipated that "data saturation" would be achieved with two life history case studies. Each individual life narrative was intended to present a unique story that could elucidate the meaning of suicidal behavior and masculinity to those individuals who enacted it. The two life stories could be suggestive of wider patterns of suicidal behavior. Messerschmidt (1999) undertook life history interviews with two men who had engaged in violent crime and made tentative suggestions toward a new theory for understanding violent criminal offenders. I drew parallels between the two life histories, which allowed for some comparison between the two cases and mirrored, to a lesser extent, the detailed process of collective analysis that was later conducted with 18 participants.

CONCLUSION

The suicide literature supports an association between male suicide and social factors such as employment status, relationship breakdown, and lack of supportive relationships (Gunnell, Middleton, Whitley, Dorling, & Frankel, 2003; McDowell, 2003; Smalley et al., 2005). The actual mechanism of this association had rarely been investigated and remained uncertain. Life histories, underpinned by a gender relations framework, revealed a method particularly relevant to the examination of male suicide. The method takes us beyond simple statistical associations between suicide and social factors and allows a deeper understanding of the relationship between gender and suicidal behavior. These theorized life histories were able to confirm and expand on the work of Anne Cleary (2005). Whereas Cleary's work specifically demonstrated that hegemonic masculinity was the link between male suicide and help-seeking behavior, the theorized life history methodology pointed to the influence of masculinity in the choice of the suicide method and made visible the complex interplay between masculinities and other social institutions.

The findings detail the mechanism of masculinity in male suicide and the way this mediates between other social factors such as marital breakdown and employment status. They describe how dominant depictions of masculinity curtail emotional expression and influence the choice of the suicide method. The findings from this study form an honors thesis (Dunn, 2008).

They have been presented at an international conference (paper available online; River & Fisher, 2010). The preliminary findings of the larger study of 18 men are outlined in the *Australian Nursing Journal* (River, 2012).

REFERENCES

Ashe, F. (2007). *The new politics of masculinity: Men, power and resistance*. London, UK: Routledge.

Canetto, S. S., & Sakinofsky, I. (1998). The gender paradox in suicide. *Suicide and Life—Threatening Behavior, 28*(1), 1–23.

Carrigan, T., Connell, R., & Lee, J. (1985). Toward a new sociology of masculinity. *Theory and Sociology, 14,* 551–604.

Cleary, A. (2005). Death rather than disclosure: Struggling to be a real man. *Irish Journal of Sociology, 14*(2), 155–176.

Connell, P. (1987). Teaching language form, meaning, and function to specific-language-impaired children. In S. Rosenberg (ed.), *Advances in applied psycholinguistics, Volume I: First-language development* (pp. 40–75). New York, NY: Cambridge University Press.

Connell, R. W. (1998). Reply to Patricia Yancey Martin and Judith Lorber. *Gender and Society 12*(4), 474–477.

Connell, R. W. (2000). *The men and the boys*. Sydney, Australia: Allen and Unwin.

Connell, R. W. (2002). *Gender*. Cambridge: Polity Press.

Connell, R. W. (2005). *Masculinities* (2nd ed.). Sydney, Australia: Allen and Unwin.

Connell, R. W. (2010). Lives of businessmen. Reflection on life-history and contemporary hegemonic masculinity. *Österreichische Zeitschrift für Soziologie, 35*(2), 54–71.

Connell, R. W., & Messerschmidt, J. W. (2005). Hegemonic masculinity: Rethinking the concept. *Gender and Society, 19*(6), 829–859.

Donaldson, M., & Poynting, S. (2007). *Ruling class men: Money, sex, power*. Bern, Switzerland: Peter Lang.

Dowsett, G. (1996) *Practicing desire: Homosexual sex in the era of AIDS*. Stanford, CA: Stanford University Press.

Dunn, J. (2008). *Dying to be a man: Towards an understanding of the relationship between masculinity and male suicidal behaviour* (Unpublished Bachelor of Nursing [Honours] thesis). Sydney, Australia: The University of Sydney.

Elnour, A. A., & Harrison, J. (2008). Lethality of suicide methods. *Injury Prevention, 14,* 39–45.

Fisher, M. J. (2006). *Masculinities and men in nursing: An exploratory survey and life history study* (Unpublished doctoral thesis). University of Sydney, Australia.

Fisher, M. J. (2009). 'Being a Chameleon': Labour processes of male nurses performing body work. *Journal of Advanced Nursing, 65*(12), 2668–2677.

Fisher, M. J., & Chilko, N. (2012). Gender and obesity. In L. Baur, S. Twigg, & S. Magnusson, (Eds.), *A modern epidemic—Expert perspectives on obesity and diabetes*. Sydney, NSW: Sydney University Press.

Gallagher, R., Marshall, A., & Fisher, M. J. (2010). Women's symptoms and treatment seeking behaviour in their first acute coronary syndrome. *Heart and Lung: The Journal of Acute and Critical Care, 39*(6), 477–484.

Gallagher, R., Marshall, A., Fisher, M. J., & Elliott, D., (2008). On my own; Experiences of recovery from acute coronary syndrome for women living alone. *Heart and Lung: The Journal of Acute and Critical Care, 37*(6), 417–424.

Gunnell, D. J., Middleton, N., Whitley, E., Dorling, D., & Frankel, S. (2003). Why are suicide rates rising in young men but falling in the elderly?—A time series analysis of trends in England and Wales 1950–1998. *Social Science and Medicine, 57*, 595–611.

Jaworski, K. (2007). *The gender of suicide.* Unpublished Doctor of Philosophy thesis, University of South Australia.

Kimmel, M. (1994). Masculinity as homophobia: Fear, shame and silence in the construction of gender identity. In H. Brod & M. Kaufman (Eds.). *Theorizing masculinities.* Thousand Oaks, CA: Sage.

Mann, J. J. (2002). A current perspective of suicide and attempted suicide. *Annals of Internal Medicine, 136*(4), 302–311.

McDowell, M. (2003). *Redundant masculinities? Employment change and white working class youth.* Carlton, VIC: Blackwell.

Messerschmidt, J. W. (1999). Making bodies matter: Adolescent masculinities, the body and varieties of violence. *Theoretical Criminology, 3*(2), 197–220.

Messerschmidt, J. W. (2000). *Nine lives: Adolescent masculinities, the body, and violence.* Boulder, CO: Westview Press.

Messner, M. (1995). *Power at play: Sports and the problem of masculinity.* Boston, MA: Beacon Press.

Miller, R. L. (2000). *Researching life stories and family histories.* London, UK: Sage.

Page, A., Morrell, S., Taylor, R., Dudley, M., & Carter, G. (2007). Further increases in rural suicide in young Australian adults: Secular trends, 1979–2003. *Social Science and Medicine, 65*(3), 442–453.

Plummer, K. (2001). *Documents of life: An invitation to a critical humanism.* London, UK: Sage.

Psychiatry Online. (2008, April 8). DSM-IV-TR: Major depressive episode [Online], Retrieved from http://psychiatryonline.org/guidelines.aspx

River, J. (2012). Suicidal masculinities: Understanding the gendered nature of male suicide. *Australian Nursing Journal, 20*(5), 49.

River, J., & Fisher, M. (2010, November). Dying to be a man: Towards an understanding of the relationship between masculinity and male suicidal behaviour. Making sense of suicide: 1st Global Conference, Probing the Boundaries, Interdisciplinary Net, Prague, Czech Republic.

Schofield, T., Connell, R. W., Walker, L., Wood, J., & Butland, D. L. (2000). Understanding men's health and illness: A gender-relations approach to policy, research, and practice. *Journal of American College Health, 47*, 247–256.

Schofield, T., & Goodwin, S. (2006). Gender politics and public policy making: Prospects for advancing gender equality. *Policy and Society, 24*(4), 23–29.

Smalley, N., Scourfield, J., & Greenland, K. (2005). Young people, gender and suicide. *Journal of Social Work, 5*(2), 133–154.

Talseth, A.G., Lindseth, A., Jacobsson, L., & Norberg, A. (1999). The meaning of suicidal in-patients' Experiences of being cared for by mental health nurses. *Journal of Advanced Nursing, 29*(5), 1034–1041.

Tatz, C. (2005). *Aboriginal suicide is different: A portrait of life and self-destruction* (2nd ed.). Canberra, Australia: Aboriginal Studies Press.

Taylor, R., Page, A., Morrell, S., Harrison, J., & Carter, G. (2005a). Social and psychiatric influences on urban-rural differentials in Australian suicide. *Suicide and Life-Threatening Behavior, 35*(3), 277–290.

Taylor, R., Page, A., Morrell, S., Harrison, J., & Carter, G. (2005b). Mental health and socio-economic variations in Australian suicide. *Social Science and Medicine, 61,* 1551–1559.

Wharton, A. S. (2005). *The sociology of gender: An introduction to theory and research,* Oxford, UK: Blackwell.

World Health Organization (WHO). (2009). Women and suicide in rural China. *Bulletin of the World Health Organization, 87*(12), 885–964. Retrieved May 5, 2014, from http://www.who.int/bulletin/volumes/87/12/09-011209/en/

CHAPTER EIGHT

USING LIFE HISTORY TO EXPLORE THE EXPERIENCE OF WOMEN LIVING WITH A RARE CHRONIC ILLNESS: LYMPHANGIOLEIOMYOMATOSIS

Denise Haylen and Murray J. Fisher

*T*his chapter examines the life history method in relation to the study of women's experiences of living with a rare chronic illness. A life history study was conducted on the experience of women living with lymphangi-oleiomyomatosis (LAM) over a life course. This study was undertaken to fulfill the requirements of a PhD by Denise Haylen and supervised by Dr. Murray Fisher. Both student and supervisor were responsible for the design of the study, but the data collection and analysis were undertaken by Denise Haylen. Life history interviews were conducted with 19 women aged 33 to 64 years. The life stories were analyzed using a modified version of Rosenthal's (1993) method of narrative analysis. The method, including decision making related to the study design and data analysis and challenges concerning recruitment, data collection, and ethical issues, is discussed in this chapter.

BACKGROUND

This life history study set out to explore the lived experience of women with LAM over a life course. LAM is a rare, chronic, incurable, systemic condition associated with progressive cystic lung disease and lymphatic and abdominal tumors (Taveira-DaSilva & Moss, 2012, p. 267). It affects women almost exclusively and often during their childbearing years. The prevalence of LAM is 3 to 5 per million people worldwide and can affect women of all races and economic backgrounds (LAM Foundation, 2013). There is a high level of variability clinically and in the rate of progression of LAM

(Cohen, Pollock-BarZiv, & Johnson, 2005, p. 879; Johnson, 1999, p. 255). Disease progression ranges from very aggressive with rapid decline in lung function to slow progress with a gradual loss of lung function over decades before interfering with activities of daily living and requiring oxygen therapy (Taveira-DaSilva, Pacheco-Rodriguez, & Moss, 2010, p. 15). Delays in diagnosis are common (Johnson, 1999, p. 256). The Multicentre International LAM Efficacy of Sirolimus (MILES) Trial, conducted 2006 to 2010, reported that sirolimus, an immunosuppressive medication, stabilized lung function and was associated with improved symptoms and quality of life related to LAM (McCormack et al., 2011, p. 1595). However, this treatment is not suitable for or available to all women with LAM and, for many women with LAM, oxygen therapy and eventually lung transplantation may be the only treatment options.

Literature Review

A literature review was conducted prior to designing the study to locate and analyze the available literature on LAM and, in particular, the lived experience of women with this condition (Haylen, Fisher, & Lawler, 2009). The literature was also reviewed for any research on the experience of living with a rare disease. A search of CINAHL, MedLine, and PsycINFO databases revealed that all research conducted into LAM to date has been quantitative scientific research. The literature was mainly descriptive and consisted largely of reviews of clinical data, larger retrospective observational studies, case studies, and presentation of genetic and cellular research and reports of clinical trials related to LAM. In nursing literature, there were two references only, both case reports, one of which was in Chinese (McCowan & Moore, 1992; Sung, Jong, & Lu, 2006). Four studies in the biomedical literature highlighted areas related to the experience of living with LAM such as quality of life (Ryu et al., 2006), subjective assessment of respiratory function (Pollock-BarZiv, Cohen, Maclean, & Downey, 2005) and management of pneumothorax (Young et al., 2006), and dyspnea and fatigue (Cohen et al., 2005). One personal account of living with LAM (Carel, 2008) was located by word of mouth but could not be found in the databases and so would not easily be located by health professionals investigating LAM. Only two studies were found on the experience of living with a rare disease: a phenomenological study ($n = 12$) on the experience of living with mycosis fungoides (Vitale, 2005) and a focus group study ($n = 4$, $n = 9$) exploring the experience of living with scleroderma as a rare disease (Joachim & Acorn, 2003).

No literature examined in depth the patient experience of LAM as a rare, chronic, incurable condition, and there was a paucity of literature exploring the experience of living with a rare disease. In response, this study proposed to use a life history methodology to explore in depth the subjective views of women with LAM and aimed to increase knowledge of the experience of living with LAM, improve the understanding of how the rarity of the disease affects the illness experience, and identify needs of women with LAM and how support might be provided for these individuals.

Significance of the Study

Although LAM is a rare disease, increasing numbers of women are being diagnosed with the condition. As a rare disease it is not uncommon for health professionals caring for these patients to have not heard of LAM or know very little about the disease and its impact on this group of patients. Examining women's subjective views of their disease provides accessible information for health professionals to increase their understanding of LAM from the patient perspective. This, in turn, enhances cooperative decision making and may improve clinical outcomes and quality of life for these women (Pollock-BarZiv et al., 2005, p. 902; Young et al., 2006, p. 1268). Improving knowledge of women's perspectives on the experience of living with LAM may also provide insights into the experience of women living with other respiratory conditions and people living with other rare diseases.

METHODOLOGY

Design

The life history method was chosen as the most suitable method for the study because of its holistic nature and focus on human experience from the viewpoint of the particular individual (Denzin, 2009, p. 220). As a chronic condition, LAM may occupy a significant portion of a woman's life. Time and context, therefore, are important aspects of the research question. In studying lives, life history allows the exploration of experience over time in the context of a whole life, including both the individual social context and the broader historical context. Life history examines events and how they impact an individual woman and her life trajectory, revealing turning points, epiphanies, and transformations that may occur over the course of living with LAM. It provides a way of understanding the meaning of the illness experience for individuals and how meaning might change over time.

Life history method has been used in studies that have linked individual lives with culture and broader historical and social issues in a range of disciplines such as sociology, education, psychology, psychiatry, women's studies, gerontology, health promotion, and occupational therapy (Cole & Knowles, 2001, p. 12). It has been infrequently used to examine chronic illness experience (Admi, 1995a, 1995b, 1996; Admi & Shaman, 2007; Stamm et al., 2008).

Analysis in life history is a challenging process as there are no clear cut guidelines to follow. The process has been recognized as difficult to describe, creative, convoluted, chaotic, and time consuming (Cole & Knowles, 2001, p. 99; Plummer, 2001, pp. 152, 166). A number of analytical approaches have been adopted across the various disciplines, including grounded theory (Admi, 1995a, 1995b, 1996; Admi & Shaman, 2007; Strauss & Glaser, 1977), analytic induction (Becker, 1963), Sartre's progressive-regressive method (Denzin, 1987), structural analysis of gender relations (Connell, 1995), narrative analysis (Polkinghorne, 1995; Price-Lackey, 1996), analysis of lives for dimensions, turnings, and adaptations (Mandelbaum, 1973), and the biographical interpretative approach (Jones, 2001; Jones & Rupp, 2000; King & Chamberlayne, 1996; Rosenthal, 1993).

In deciding which approach to adopt for analysis, two aspects of the process were considered: the representativeness of the cases and the level of interpretation to be undertaken (Plummer, 2001). Plummer (2001, p. 153) notes that life history research provides understanding and insights into the topic of research rather than generalizations and explanations. The exploratory nature of this life history study and the rarity of LAM were factors influencing the choice of the analytic procedure. The particular purpose of this study was to understand the range of experience of living with LAM and to allow women's subjective views to be heard. It was less concerned with providing a general theory of the experience of living with LAM or living with a rare disease than with generating insights by exploring in detail the experiences of women of different ages, cultural and social backgrounds, and at different stages of the disease. The cases studied could, however, be linked to broader chronic illness experience through their examination in relation to existing theories (Chamberlayne, Bornat, & Wengraf, 2000, p. 22; Plummer, 2001, p. 159).

The level of interpretation to be undertaken was the second factor to consider in choosing an analytic procedure. Plummer (2001, pp. 179, 180) suggests "a continuum of 'construction'" in relation to interpretation. The unedited life history stands at one end of the continuum. Here the participant's life story is not interpreted and speaks for itself. At the other end of the continuum is the researcher's theoretical construction made independent of the participant's account. In between, constructions range from edited personal documents, systematic thematic analysis in which participants speak for themselves but have their accounts organized around themes and linked to theory, and researcher-imposed interpretation of the data verified by examples. In relation to this life history study, it was important not only to preserve the voice of participants but also to interpret the accounts to provide deeper levels of meaning and understanding. I decided that the level of interpretation of a systematic thematic analysis as part of the analytic procedure was appropriate for meeting the goals of the study.

The biographic interpretive method, using a narrative approach and an adaptation of Rosenthal's (1993) hermeneutic case reconstruction, provided the framework for data collection and analysis for this study owing to its strong ability to explore the personal meaning of the illness experience for women and its impact on their personal biographies (Chamberlayne et al., 2000, p. 9).

Hermeneutics using Gadamer's approach formed the philosophical background to the study. Gadamer's philosophical hermeneutics holds that "understanding occurs in interpreting" and that "language is the universal medium in which understanding occurs" (Gadamer, 1975/2004, p. 390). A central tenet of Gadamer's philosophy was the concept of prejudice. For Gadamer (1975/2004, p. 278), the prejudices of an individual are their background understandings—that of the family, society, and state in which one lives. These prejudices form a person's historical being and always influence any experience, interaction, or interpretation. In the context of a narrative biographical interview, the narrator and researcher bring their prejudices and prior perspectives to the interaction and interpretation of the life story. This is acknowledged as part of the interactions of the narrators with their social world (Rosenthal, 1993, p. 65). Narrator, researcher, and reader of the research are all situated within the "hermeneutic circle of interpretation" (Sandelowski, 1991, p. 62).

Sample

Originally, I proposed to use purposive sampling for this study. In the context of a rare disease I sought participants of varying ages, social and cultural backgrounds, and at different stages of the disease to give as broad a range as possible of the experience of living with LAM. In accordance with the Human Research Ethics Committee's (HREC) approval, a medical gatekeeper at a hospital that provided a clinic for LAM patients agreed to send out invitations to potential participants to join the study. It was requested that potential participants were purposively selected. However, the medical gatekeeper, used to scientific quantitative research and less familiar with qualitative research, felt this would introduce "bias" to the study and, without consultation, issued invitations randomly. Over a period of 3 months, only five participants consented to join the study.

Additional local issues representing broader concerns for nursing research impacted the recruitment process. Recruitment was delayed by 2 weeks owing to unexpected political issues related to medical "ownership" of patients and a perception that the research was competing with another scientific study related to the same population. A complaint was made to the HREC by a physician who was concerned that patients attending the public hospital clinic and who were, therefore, considered to be under the hospital's care, had been recruited to the study without prior approval of the hospital. A second concern was that participation in the life history study would interfere with a concurrent clinical trial in which some patients were also participating. The matter was resolved following HREC review by a change to the research protocol, whereby, within the hospital, individual physicians would be notified of the study and, at their own discretion, would choose to invite potential participants to join the study. Recruitment was dependent on the preferences of the medical gatekeepers. The situation illustrates how power structures within health care settings, in which patients are perceived to be "owned" by medicine, can reduce the autonomy of nursing research. Despite being a registered nurse at the hospital, in this hierarchical context, my qualitative nursing study, although it had received relevant ethics approval and was unrelated to any medical activities, was subject to medical supervision. Rather than collaborating to plan recruitment, I was required to comply with the preferences of medical gatekeepers. On reflection, I realized I could have bypassed the medical gatekeepers and, instead, applied initially for HREC approval to recruit directly through the patient organization.

It was decided that it was necessary to find alternative means of recruitment. Following a further delay in having the necessary amendment approved by the HREC, the patient organization in Australia, LAM Australasia Research Alliance (LARA), was contacted for assistance. The women were pleased that someone was taking an interest in their rare condition. I presented the aim and design of the study to a meeting of some members of LARA, and they indicated their support. Recruitment then became a process of network sampling, as members of LARA networked within the organization to inform members of the study. Through this process a further 14 women consented to join the study. Nineteen participants in total were recruited to join the study over a period of 8 months.

Although I had been unable to sample purposively, I did, in fact, achieve the aim of recruiting participants with a broad range of experience of LAM. The 19 women participating in the study ranged in age from 33 to 64 years, had been diagnosed with LAM from between 18 months and 15 years, and came from a range of cultural backgrounds including Australian, Scandinavian, South American, East European, Greek, Asian, and British.

Ethical Considerations

Ethics approval for the study was granted by the HREC of a city hospital and was ratified by the ethics committee of the university at which I am a doctoral candidate. All participants were over 18 years of age and spoke English. They received a Participant Information and Consent Form, which informed them in a clear and easily understood manner of the nature, aims, and process of the research project and that they could withdraw consent at any time without any penalty and without their care being affected in any way. Participants freely gave their consent to be interviewed and to have their medical records accessed before being interviewed. When participant consents had been received, ethics approval to access medical records also had to be sought from three other hospitals attended by some participants.

Audiotapes and transcripts were available only to me and my two university supervisors. During the research process, data were stored on a password-protected computer. At the completion of the study the research data were deleted from the computer, and audio recordings and transcripts were then located in a locked cupboard in a university office, where they will be stored for 7 years and then destroyed.

An ethical consideration in conducting research with a small group in the context of a rare disease is that some participants were known to each other, and particular care had to be taken with de-identification of the data. This was achieved through the use of pseudonyms and changing or generalizing identifying details such as nationality (e.g., Asian rather than Chinese), location (e.g., urban or regional rather than a specific state or city), and occupation. Particular caution was taken in the presentation of the life histories. Interpretations will be presented collectively for public publications rather than as complete individual life histories so that individual lives are not identifiable.

Whole transcripts and interpretations were not returned to the participants. This decision was made in keeping with the underlying assumption of life history research that the life story told at the time of the interview is true for the narrator at that time and that, later, meaning may change in the light of new experiences (Plummer, 2001, p. 239; Sandelowski, 1993, p. 5). This is also consistent with the hermeneutic view that, as a story is told, the horizon of the past is fused with the horizon of the present to change and enrich its meaning (Widdershoven, 1993, p. 13).

Data Collection

Data collection involved conducting two interviews with each participant as well as accessing their hospital medical records. The first interview, as per Rosenthal's (1993) method, was an open style of interview in which the participant was invited to tell the story of her life in whatever way she chose. I listened without interrupting except to give verbal signs of attentiveness. This allowed the woman to choose to narrate what she regarded were the significant aspects of her life story in her own time and manner. This style of interviewing was totally focused on the participant and her perspective and to maintain openness to her truth (Gadamer, 1975/2004, p. 271). The second interview, conducted later after initial reflection on the first interview, allowed certain issues to be discussed in greater depth and to raise topics not covered in the first interview. I found that sensitive issues were often discussed in the second interview after we had established a rapport in which the participant could feel a sense of trust and comfort with me. Interviews lasted between 49 and 240 minutes, on average between 120 and 150 minutes each.

The rarity of LAM provided challenges for data collection. The interval between the first and second interviews varied as, in the context of a rare disease, participants were located throughout Australia. Interviews had to be arranged for a time that was convenient to participants and when I was able to travel to the relevant locations. Many of the participants were working or had other responsibilities or commitments that influenced scheduling of the second interview.

Traveling long distances to five states of Australia to conduct 35 interviews was time consuming and costly. I attended the medical record departments of four hospitals located in four different states to access participants' medical records and took notes by hand. Although long-distance interviews could alternatively have been conducted by phone or Skype, I felt it was important to honor each woman's story by being personally present with her. This facilitated the building of excellent rapport with each participant and rich data collection.

Interviews were conducted at a time and place convenient to each participant. The majority of the interviews were conducted in the homes of participants. Two interviews took place in hotel rooms, two in a private office of a workplace, and one in a closed office of a university. Each of these settings was quiet and private. One interview was conducted in a shopping mall and one in a cafe. These were less satisfactory owing to the less private nature of the settings and the level of background noise.

Each interview was transcribed verbatim and de-identified as transcribed. Initially I transcribed two interviews personally, but the length of time taken for this was prohibitive for the transcribing of 35 long interviews in the time allocated to a doctoral thesis. The remainder were, therefore, transcribed professionally, a factor that added additional cost to the conduct of the study but reduced time delays.

Data Analysis

Rosenthal's (1993) biographic interpretive method, the hermeneutic case reconstruction, was modified to analyze the data. The unit of analysis was the life story of each woman as represented by her whole narrative, told at the time of the interview and transcribed verbatim. Each woman's medical record was also examined. For each case, the process of analyzing the data was carried out in three stages—construction of the biographical account of the life, analysis of the life story, and reconstruction of the life history. Each case was analyzed individually before comparisons and contrasts were made across cases.

Whereas Rosenthal (1993, p. 61) believes that life history and life story are "continuously and dialectically linked and produce each other," she distinguishes between life story and life history. The life story is narrated and constructed in the present moment (Rosenthal, 2002, p. 178). Life history is defined by Rosenthal (2002, p. 178) as "the experiences that a person has lived through." The life story forms the "data base" from which the life history can be reconstructed. In this process experiences are reconstructed in the chronological sequence in which they occurred (Rosenthal, 1993, pp. 60, 61). The reconstructed life history represents the past perspective and "the biographical meaning that the experiences had at the time they happened" (Rosenthal, 1993, p. 69). Rosenthal (1993, p. 61, 2002, p. 178) sees the reconstruction of the life story and the life history as a "hermeneutic case reconstruction," and both are interpretations.

The biographical account was constructed to represent the objective facts of a woman's life and the trajectory of her illness. These included the facts documented in her medical record, including background and biomedical information, and those facts narrated in the life story that were free of interpretation. They were extracted from notes taken from the medical record and from the life story as told at the time of the interviews. This information was then constructed in chronological sequence to show the objective process of the illness trajectory. The biographical account provided a background of events and processes to which the narrated life story could be compared to show which of this data was selected for narration, in what order, and their relative significance (Rosenthal, 1993, p. 68).

The second stage of analysis in Rosenthal's (1993) method of hermeneutic case reconstruction is the thematic field analysis. The narrated life story represents "a sequence of mutually interrelated themes," and the thematic field is defined as "the sum of events or situations presented in connection with the theme that forms the background or horizon against which the theme stands out as the central focus" (Rosenthal, 1993, p. 64). Analysis involves a complex process of text sequentialization whereby small sequences of text are interpreted in order through the generation and testing of hypotheses (Rosenthal, 1993, p. 70).

Rosenthal's process of thematic field analysis was modified for this study for the following reasons. First, Rosenthal's (1993, p. 70) aim of the thematic field analysis to "interpret the nature and function of the presentation in the interview and not the biographical experiences themselves" was not the primary aim of this study, which sought to understand the meaning of illness experience. Rosenthal's method was directed at understanding the meaning of wartime experiences during the National Socialist era in Germany. In this context, a narrator's motivations for decision making and action in the past may be hidden from their consciousness as a coping mechanism or because they wish to present themselves differently in the present in line with their present perspectives. Rosenthal's method was a way to uncover and interpret these hidden meanings. In contrast, this study was focused on understanding the participants' perspectives on their experiences and, through interpretation, develop deeper levels of meaning rather than uncover hidden agendas.

Second, Rosenthal's method of sequential analysis, concerned mainly with structure and representation, was very prescribed, rigid, and difficult to undertake with a number of cases in the time allotted to a doctoral thesis conducted by a single researcher. It lacked flexibility and room for creativity. Similar concerns were expressed by Jones (2004, p. 50), who modified the biographical interpretive approach in a study of identity and the informal care role in 2001 (Jones, 2001) by reducing strict adherence to text structure sequentialization to allow a more creative approach to data analysis. I decided that the process of sequential analysis would not provide meaningful interpretations in the context of this study, which is concerned with illness experience. Rosenthal's method was, therefore, modified at this stage of the analysis by choosing thematic analysis as the most suitable method to analyze the life story. This decision was also congruent with the earlier decision made regarding the level of interpretation to be undertaken in the study.

Thematic analysis has been used with narrative and biographical approaches (Fischer, 1982; Reissman, 2008; Williams, 1984). The data are searched for themes that, through interpretation by the researcher, uncover participant meanings (Saldana, 2013, p. 177). Thematic analysis is focused on the content of the text. Stories are identified and analyzed intact in longer sequences, and attention is paid to time and context (Reissman, 2008, p. 74). Analyzing stories in the context of the whole text and the whole life preserves the gestalt of the biography in the sense of the underlying structure of personal meaning, which guided the selection of stories as narrated in each interview (Cole & Knowles, 2001, p. 119; Rosenthal, 1993, p. 62). These features of thematic analysis and its holistic and interpretive nature suited the analysis of the life stories and were congruent with the underlying hermeneutic philosophy of the study and Rosenthal's method (Rosenthal, 1993, p. 87). The approach taken in the study was inductive, in that themes came directly from the data (Ryan & Bernard, 2003, p. 88). Theory was applied to the interpreted themes to see their relationship to broader concerns.

In conducting a thematic analysis of the life stories I first read, reread, and reflected on the text. Words and phrases that seemed significant and provided insights were highlighted (Sandelowski, 1995, p. 373). Biographical facts and the objective facts of the illness experience were extracted for the biographical accounts. The structure of the text was examined to identify which segments of text were narrations or stories. These were identified as those segments of text in which the participant told a story and elaborated on an experience or event (Rosenthal, 1993, p. 69). They were generally longer sequences, and some evaluation of the episode was involved. In contrast some sequences were reports about events without elaboration. This initial phase of analysis provided the framework for more interpretive levels of analysis (Cole & Knowles, 2001, p. 117).

Second, I analyzed the narrative sequences intact, paying attention to their context in relation to the whole text, their temporal ordering within the text, and their relationship to the initially highlighted words and phrases. The sequences were read more deeply to search for emerging patterns of meaning or themes (Cole & Knowles, 2001, p. 116; Denzin, 1989, p. 56). In particular, turning points, critical events or epiphanies were identified. They are organizing constructs by which fundamental changes in meaning are conveyed within a life story (Cole & Knowles, 2001, p. 120; Denzin, 1989, p. 70). The biographical account was compared to the life story to correlate the objective medical perspective with the woman's personal views and to see which events she had chosen to present in what sequence and their relative significance.

The narrative sequences were also scrutinized for other features that identified themes. Repetition of topics, use of metaphors and connecting words and phrases such as "because," "if," and "then," and transitions indicated by pauses and changes in content or voice tone can all signify meaning in an interview (Ryan & Bernard, 2003, p. 90). In addition, attention was paid to the significance of topics that might have been avoided (Ryan & Bernard, 2003, p. 92).

This process of identifying themes was carried out by hand with a hard copy of the text. Meaningful words and phrases and narrative segments were highlighted in the transcript. Initial responses to the themes were noted in the margins. Long periods of reflection were involved to grasp deeper levels of meaning and allow themes to further develop. I felt this method kept me immersed in the individual life and the data within the transcript, avoided fracturing the data, and kept a sense of the whole narrative and the context of individual stories within it. It also enhanced intuitive and creative responses, which are a feature of life history research (Cole & Knowles, 2001, p. 102; Plummer, 2001, p. 152).

The descriptive identification of themes was followed by a more interpretive analysis of the themes. This process was not necessarily linear but often iterative with deeper levels of interpretation emerging at different stages of reflection (Wolcott, 1994, p. 11). As themes developed, a folder for each theme was created in which themes were named and described in detail. This maintained consistency in the meanings interpreted within each case and across cases. Interpretations remained grounded in the text and relevant quotes representing the themes were selected. Interpretations matured with reflection and writing over time. Part of the reflective process involved personal reflection on how the context of the interview, my relationship with the participant, and my own life experiences and professional knowledge influenced the interpretation. The process was hermeneutic.

Mind mapping was used to plot themes visually. This allowed the analysis to be visualized and connections and differences between themes to be identified and interpreted. Mind mapping reflects the radiant thinking process of the brain and, through its expanding branches, encourages new and creative associations to be made within and across the branches

(Buzan & Buzan, 2010, p. 31). This facilitated the interpretation of deeper levels of meaning through the linking of themes into more abstract concepts and overarching themes pertaining to the life and illness experience. In addition it provided a visual record of the process of interpretation, which added to the rigor of the analysis. Developing interpretations were checked and agreed on within the supervisory team.

Theory was used at the interpretive stage of the analysis. Interpreted themes were examined in the light of existing theories to extend the analysis and link the particulars of the unique case to broader issues and more general knowledge (Wolcott, 1994, p. 43). The meanings interpreted from the individual case have the potential to extend theoretical perspectives. From a hermeneutic perspective, the analysis at this stage could be regarded as a "hermeneutic of questioning," in which interpretations were questioned in relation to theory, as opposed to a "hermeneutic of empathy," in which the aim of interpretation was to understand the experience from the participant's perspective (Smith, Flowers, & Larkin, 2009, p. 36).

Analysis of the life story was complete when no new themes emerged. The life history was then reconstructed. In this process, the biographical account was merged with the interpreted life story to present the life and illness experience in chronological order and show how meaning had changed over time. The life history was the product of the participant's subjective interpretation of her life and my interpretation of her life story as told. The life history was therefore co-constructed.

A double hermeneutic is present, as the meaning of the past experience of the participant was fused with her present perspective in the life story told in our interaction. That meaning was fused with my interpretation of the text filtered through my own perspectives. Applying Gadamer's theory of interpretation, understanding was enriched through this "fusion of horizons" (Gadamer, 1975/2004, p. 305). The concept of the hermeneutic circle is also present. Analysis of the life story involved moving between narrative segments and themes as parts and the life story as a whole. Reconstructing the life history brought together the objective facts, subjective life story, and interpreted themes as parts to form a whole, the new text of the life history, providing enriched understanding.

When each individual case had been analyzed, analysis was conducted across cases. Each case and its themes were plotted on a mind map so that relationships between themes could be identified. Some themes could be grouped together in higher order themes, which could further illuminate individual cases. Areas of difference between cases were also analyzed.

In this way, shared qualities of women's experiences of living with LAM as well as unique features could be presented (Smith, Flowers, & Larkin, 2009, p. 101). Further examination of these qualities against the literature related to living with chronic illness and a rare disease, and current theoretical perspectives gave a more generalized perspective of the women's particular experiences of living with LAM to add to the understanding of illness experience.

Rigor

Rigor was maintained in this study by adopting a transparent framework for conducting the study and a systematic approach to the analysis of the data. The procedures and decision making involved were reflected on and clearly expressed. The use of mind mapping documented and demonstrated how interpretations were made. These processes provided an audit trail for readers of the research. Rigor was also associated with articulating ethical awareness and reflexivity in regard to my own role as researcher, the intersubjective relationship between me and each participant, and the impact of these on the research process and knowledge production (Davies & Dodd, 2002, p. 285; Roulston, 2010, p. 116).

Anna's Life History

What I thought my life would be like and what it's like are two whole different stories. (Anna, 2009)

Anna's life history was constructed as a single case for an honor's thesis (Haylen, 2009) before undertaking the larger life history study. Anna was a 35-year-old woman who had been living with LAM for 11 years at the time of our interviews. She experienced her first symptom, a spontaneous lung collapse, when she was 23 years old but was not diagnosed for another 2 years. Anna's case demonstrates how the life history can be constructed around critical events and turning points. These life-altering experiences revealed decision-making processes, personal identity and agency, and transformations as she constructed her health while living with LAM as a chronic illness. This was an effective way to uncover the personal meaning of the illness for Anna and changes in meaning over time. A mind map shows the development of themes and the construction of Anna's life history around the critical events and turning points in her illness experience (see Figure 8.1).

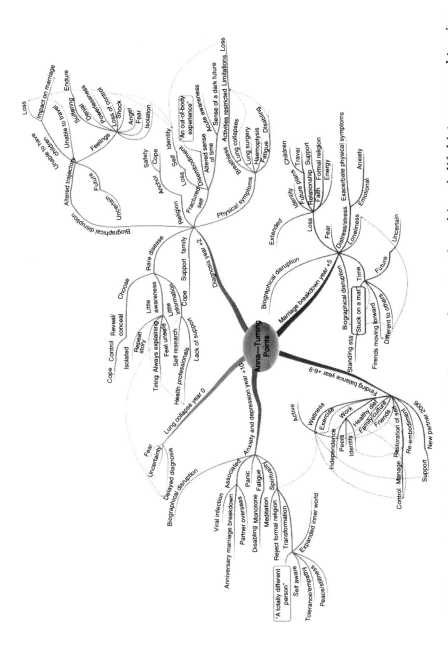

Figure 8.1 *Mind map showing the development of themes and construction of Anna's life history around turning points and critical events in her illness experience.*

183

Drawing on the work of Bury (1982), Anna's life history represented her life with LAM as a series of biographical disruptions. These created a process of biographical transformation influenced by the social context of her illness experience and the rarity of LAM. Three periods of transformation were identified:

1. The critical events of diagnosis and marriage breakdown associated with disembodiment and a sense of loss and isolation

   I literally felt like my whole world fell apart . . . . For the first time in my life I have no control over what's happening in my life . . . . It was almost like an out of body experience, 'cause I was looking at myself, in a sense going this is not really happening 'cause I'm only 25, and this can't be happening. (Anna, 2009, on being diagnosed with LAM)

   It was too much for me in the sense of having to deal with not being well but . . . that was a double blow because all of this stuff was happening within a 2-year period . . . . I literally felt like my whole world fell apart, from my health, my whole life, the person I'm beginning to build a life with . . . . I think what happens emotionally and mentally to anyone, to me in particular, is far worse than what's going on physically. (Anna, 2009, on the breakup of her marriage 2 years after diagnosis)

2. A stable period after a turning point of divorce associated with reembodiment, restoration of the self and balance

   My job's important to me and having that financial independence and financial income . . . just all those aspects of your life, trying to keep it balanced . . . not tax myself too much or wear myself thin . . . . It's good to have that option to be able to do a bit of work at home so I still feel like me.

3. The third critical event of severe anxiety and depression associated with a deepened spirituality and expanded inner world

   The sense of it [LAM] being something that's life threatening and something that makes you stop, you ponder about all these things, about life, and you know I've gone beyond the "what if's," so more about just focusing inwards and what can I do to look after my spirit, look after my mind and my inner sense of being.

Anna's case has been presented at an international conference (Haylen, Fisher, & Patching, 2011). The findings of the larger study will be disseminated by presenting at national and international medical, nursing, and LAM-related conferences, and in health care settings, which women with LAM may attend. They will also be published in peer-reviewed journals.

SUMMARY

Life history in the research of chronic illness experience reflects the complexity of the human experience it is examining. It can only access the life as told at the time of the interview, and meaning will continue to change for a person with new experiences as the illness progresses and social circumstances change. It would take a longitudinal study to map experience over the total life. However, although there are many challenges, life history is able to capture multiple aspects of the chronic illness experience, including the biological, physical effect of the illness; personal meaning and social contexts; and the temporal dimension of the experience. In this way, it links personal, physical, and social realities across the life course to give a more complete view of illness experience over time.

REFERENCES

Admi, H. (1995a). The life history: A viable approach to nursing research. *Nursing Research, 44*(3), 186–188.

Admi, H. (1995b). "Nothing to hide and nothing to advertise": Managing disease-related information. *Western Journal of Nursing Research, 17*(5), 484–501.

Admi, H. (1996). Growing up with a chronic health condition: A model of an ordinary lifestyle. *Qualitative Health Research, 6*(2), 163–183.

Admi, H., & Shaman, B. (2007). Living with epilepsy: Ordinary people coping with extraordinary situations. *Qualitative Health Research, 17*(9), 1178–1187.

Becker, H. S. (1963). *Outsiders: Studies in the sociology of deviance.* New York, NY: The Free Press of Glencoe.

Bury, M. (1982). Chronic illness as biographical disruption. *Sociology of Health and Illness, 4*(2), 167–182.

Buzan, T., & Buzan, B. (2010). *The mind map book unlock your creativity, boost your memory, change your life.* Harlow, Essex, UK: BBC Active.

Carel, H. (2008). *Illness.* Stocksfield, UK: Acumen.

Chamberlayne, P., Bornat, J., & Wengraf, T. (2000). The biographical turn. In P. Chamberlayne, J. Bornat, & T. Wengraf (Eds.), *The turn to biographical methods in social science comparative issues and examples*. Milton Park, UK: Routledge.

Cohen, M. M., Pollock-BarZiv, S., & Johnson, S. R. (2005). Emerging clinical picture of lymphangioleiomyomatosis. *Thorax, 60*, 875–879.

Cole, A. L., & Knowles, J. G. (2001). *Lives in context: The art of life history research*. Oxford, UK: AltaMira Press.

Connell, R. W. (1995). *Masculinities*. Cambridge, UK: Polity Press.

Davies, D., & Dodd, J. (2002). Qualitative research and the question of rigor. *Qualitative Health Research, 12*(2), 279–289.

Denzin, N. K. (1987). *The alcoholic self*. Newbury Park, CA: Sage.

Denzin, N. K. (1989). *Interpretive biography*. Newbury Park, CA: Sage.

Denzin, N. K. (2009). *The research act a theoretical introduction to sociological methods*. New Brunswick, NJ: Transaction.

Fischer, W. (1982). *Time and chronic illness. A study on social constitution of temporality*. Habilitation thesis, University of California, Berkeley.

Gadamer, H. G. (1975/2004). *Truth and method* (J. Weisheimer & D. G. Marshall, Trans.). London, UK: Continuum Publishing Group. (Original work published 1975.)

Haylen, D. (2009). *Living with lymphangioleiomyomatosis: A life history*. Unpublished Bachelor of Nursing (Honour's) thesis, The University of Sydney.

Haylen, D., Fisher, M. J., & Lawler, J. (2009). Living with lymphangioleiomyomatosis (LAM): A literature review. *Transplant Nurses Journal, 18*(3), 20–25.

Haylen, D., Fisher, M. J., & Patching, J. (2011). Using life history to explore the experience of living with a rare chronic illness, lymphangioleiomyomatosis (LAM). *International Journal of Qualitative Methods, 10*(4), 520–521. Retrieved from http://ejournals.library.ualberta.ca/index.php/IJQM/issue/view/733

Joachim, G., & Acorn, S. (2003). Life with a rare chronic disease: The scleroderma experience. *Journal of Advanced Nursing, 42*(6), 598–606.

Johnson, S. (1999). Lymphangioleiomyomatosis: Clinical features, management and basic mechanisms. *Thorax, 54*, 254–264.

Jones, C., & Rupp, S. (2000). Understanding the carers' world: A biographical-interpretive case study. In P. Chamberlayne, J. Bornat, & T. Wengraf (Eds.), *The turn to biographical methods in social science comparative issues and examples*. Milton Park, UK: Routledge.

Jones, K. (2001). *Narratives of identity and the informal care role*. Unpublished PhD thesis. De Montfort University, Leicester.

Jones, K. (2004). The turn to a narrative knowing of persons: Minimalist passive interviewing technique and team analysis of narrative qualitative data. In F. Rapport (Ed.), *New qualitative methodologies in health and social care research*. London, UK: Routledge.

King, A., & Chamberlayne, P. (1996). Comparing the informal sphere: Public and private relations of welfare in east and west Germany. *Sociology, 30*(4), 741–762.

LAM Foundation. (2013). *Understanding the epidemiology of LAM*. Retrieved from http://www.thelamfoundation.org/medical-providers/epidemiology-of-lam

Mandelbaum, D. G. (1973). The study of life history: Gandhi. *Current Anthropology, 14*(3), 177–206.

McCormack, F. X., Inoue, Y., Moss, J., Singer, L. G., Strange, C., Nakata, K., & Trapnell, B. C. (2011). Efficacy and safety of sirolimus in lymphangioleiomyomatosis. *The New England Journal of Medicine, 364*(17), 1595–1606.

McCowan, M., & Moore, J. (1992, August 2006). Case study of a patient with terminal lung disease awaiting a single lung transplant. *Nursing Monograph, 12*, 39–46.

Plummer, K. (2001). *Documents of life 2: An invitation to a critical humanism.* London, UK: Sage.

Polkinghorne, D. E. (1995). Narrative configuration in qualitative analysis. In J. A. Hatch, & R. Wisniewski (Eds.), *Life history and narrative.* Milton Park, UK: RoutledgeFalmer.

Pollock-BarZiv, S. M., Cohen, M. M., Maclean, H., & Downey, G. P. (2005). Patients' perceptions versus medical testing of function in women with lymphangioleiomyomatosis (LAM). *Respiratory Medicine, 99*, 901–909.

Price-Lackey, P. (1996). Jenny's story: Reinventing oneself through occupation and narrative configuration. *The American Journal of Occupational Therapy, 50*(4), 306–314.

Reissman, C. K. (2008). *Narrative methods for the human sciences.* Thousand Oaks, CA: Sage.

Rosenthal, G. (1993). Reconstruction of life stories: Principles of selection in generating stories for narrative biographical interviews. In R. Josselson & A. Lieblich (Eds.), *The narrative story of lives* (Vol. 1). London, UK: Sage.

Rosenthal, G. (2002). Family history: Life stories. *History of the Family, 7*, 175–182.

Roulston, K. (2010). *Reflective interviewing a guide to theory and practice.* London, UK: Sage.

Ryan, G. W., & Bernard, H. R. (2003). Techniques to identify themes. *Field Methods, 15*(1), 85–109.

Ryu, J. H., Moss, J., Beck, G. J., Lee, J. C., Brown, K. K., Chapman, J. T., & Fanburg, B. L. (2006). The NHLBI lymphangioleiomyomatosis registry characteristics of 230 patients at enrollment. *American Journal of Respiratory and Critical Care Medicine, 173*(1), 105–111.

Saldana, J. (2013). *The coding manual for qualitative researchers.* London, UK: Sage.

Sandelowski, M. (1991). Telling stories: Narrative approaches in qualitative research. *Image: Journal of Nursing Scholarship, 23*(3), 161–166.

Sandelowski, M. (1993). Rigor or rigor mortis: The problem of rigor in qualitative research. *Advances in Nursing Science, 16*(2), 1–8.

Sandelowski, M. (1995). Qualitative analysis: What it is and how to begin. *Research in Nursing and Health, 18*, 371–375.

Smith, J. A., Flowers, P., & Larkin, M. (2009). *Interpretative phenomenological analysis theory, method and research.* London, UK: Sage.

Stamm, T., Lovelock, L., Stew, G., Nell, V., Smolen, J., Jonsson, H., & Machold, K. (2008). I have mastered the challenge of living with a chronic illness: Life stories of people with rheumatoid arthritis. *Qualitative Health Research, 18*(5), 658–669.

Sung, R. P., Yong, S. Y., & Lu, P. C. (2006). Nursing experience with a lymphangioleiomyomatosis patient. *Hu Li Tsa Chih Journal of Nursing, 53*(4), 96–105.

Taveira-DaSilva, A. M., & Moss, J. (2012). Optimizing treatments for lymphangioleiomyomatosis. *Expert Reviews Respiratory Medicine, 6*(3), 267–276. doi:10.1586 /ers.12.26

Taveira-DaSilva, A. M., Pacheco-Rodriguez, G., & Moss, J. (2010). The natural history of lymphangioleiomyomatosis: Markers of severity, rate of progression and prognosis. *Lymphatic Research and Biology, 8*(1), 9–19.

Vitale, S. A. (2005). *Living with a rare disease: Mycosis fungoides.* Unpublished Doctor of Philosophy thesis, New York University.

Widdershoven, G. A. M. (1993). The story of life: Hermeneutic perspectives on the relationship between narrative and life history. In R. Josselson & A. Lieblich (Eds.), *The narrative study of lives* (Vol. 1). London, UK: Sage.

Williams, G. (1984). The genesis of chronic illness: Narrative re-construction. *Sociology of Health and Illness, 6*(2), 175–200.

Wolcott, H. F. (1994). *Transforming qualitative data: Description, analysis and interpretation.* Thousand Oaks, CA: Sage.

Young, L. R., Almoosa, K. F., Pollock-BarZiv, S. M., Coutinho, M., McCormack, F. X., & Sahn, S. A. (2006). Patient perspectives on management of pneumothorax in lymphangioleiomyomatosis. *Chest, 129*(5), 1267–1273. doi:10.1378/chest.129.5.1267

CHAPTER NINE

INTRODUCTION TO LIFE HISTORIES AS DOCTORAL CLASS ASSIGNMENT

Mary de Chesnay

PURPOSE

The purpose of the life histories collected in the following chapters is to introduce doctoral students to a methodology that is not usually covered in qualitative texts but that has applicability to the study of nursing phenomena. For this exercise, three doctoral students conducted abbreviated life history interviews as a class assignment for their course on qualitative methods. Their interviews were part of a larger study by de Chesnay on successfully overcoming adversity, for which she obtained institutional review board (IRB) approval from the university.

Life history as a design derived from ethnography is discussed extensively in the Chapters 1–3 of this volume, so the focus of the next three short chapters will be on the students' experience of doing life histories. The methodology for these life histories was developed by de Chesnay (2005) to explore how successful African Americans overcome racism and discrimination. The life histories were later expanded to include overcoming a variety of adversities and are part of an ongoing study by de Chesnay, Rassilyer-Bomers, Webb, and Peil (2008) and de Chesnay and colleagues (2012).

The first publication was a set of life histories with successful African American adults (de Chesnay, 2005). The second publication was a series of life histories conducted by master's degree students on clinical topics related to their interests. These topics were surviving colostomy surgery, multiple sclerosis, and bereavement (de Chesnay, et al., 2008). All students had access to individuals who had experienced the phenomena and who were willing to be interviewed. The third publication involved undergraduate nursing students who interviewed affluent adolescents about their experiences of substance abuse (de Chesnay et al., 2012). Interview number and length varied depending on the prior relationship with the participants.

The methodology was standardized and consisted of three parts: a genogram to obtain a picture of the family relationships, a timeline of critical events in the participant's life, and a semi-structured interview guide designed to elicit data on the nature of the participant's adversity (illness, trauma, or discrimination) and how he or she overcame the many challenges. The interview guide consisted of several general questions, but informants were encouraged to go in whichever direction they wished that gave the interviewer the best view of their experiences. Genograms and timelines are not included in the publication to protect the privacy of the key informants. Normally, a publication of a life history would include identifying information, but that was not the basis on which IRB approval had been obtained, so it would not be appropriate to publish identifying information here.

STEPS IN THE PROCESS

1. Receive orientation to the methodology.
2. Arrange interview with the key informant.
3. Review the consent document and obtain the participant's signature.
4. Conduct the interview. (The order of genogram, timeline, and interview vary and are somewhat overlapping—e.g., new events are often remembered during the interview.)
5. Analyze the interview and field notes.
6. Arrange follow-up interviews.
7. Present the results to the key informant for verification and comment.
8. Write the report of the interview(s).

Consent Process

In the three life histories in this book, the original principal investigator (PI) (de Chesnay) had obtained IRB approval, and the process was prescribed by the university. She oriented the students to the process during class to ensure they followed the university procedure for obtaining informed consent. First, the consent form was prepared by the faculty PI and then adapted by each student to fit her research questions.

Conducting the Interview

The following questions served as a general guide for the interview. I have used the example of breast cancer, but students tailored the questions for their topics and participants. The questions are not necessarily asked in order. In ethnographic interviewing of which life history can be considered a type, participants often start interviews with comments that lead the researcher in a different direction, and participants are encouraged to digress to further explain their responses.

> As I explained when I asked you to allow me to interview you, I understand that you were diagnosed with breast cancer about 15 years ago and that you are in remission. Tell me how you learned you had cancer.

> 1. What was your reaction at the time you learned you had cancer? For example, what thoughts and feelings did you have and what did you do?
> 2. How did your family learn you had cancer?
> 3. What were their reactions?
> 4. What support did you have from family, friends, health care professionals, and others?
> 5. What were the primary ways in which you coped with your illness?
> 6. What is the single most powerful force in your life that helps you cope—not only with the diagnosis of breast cancer but also the problems of daily life?
> 7. What have I not asked that you think I should have asked?

It is important to note that these questions require thoughtfulness on the part of the key informant, and it is common for them to tell stories, relate incidents, and digress while answering the interview questions. They often do not answer in order because they might start the interview in a different place than Question 1. For example, in the first study with successful African Americans, several people immediately started talking about family and church support before I even asked about their experiences growing up. One man said, "Sure I will be happy to talk to you because my pastor said you were okay and I owe him a lot." He then told a long story about how the pastor had helped him. This is actually a response to Question 4 about resources. It is critical for the researcher to listen respectfully, allow the person to go in any direction he or she chooses, and eventually get around to the other questions in the interview guide. Interviewing for any type of qualitative research requires flexibility and the ability to allow the participant or key informant to go in any direction. The burden of getting the person back on track belongs to the interviewer, but the story belongs to the informant.

Analyze Interview and Field Notes

Each student prepared a transcription of the taped interview and arranged responses according to the format of content, process, and themes or concepts. The next step was to go through the data several times by themselves to elicit the major themes and concepts of the interview. Once these were identified, the student allowed the data to gel while she thought about the results and came to conclusions.

Follow-Up

If necessary, students contacted key informants for follow-up interviews as described in their chapters. The need for this varies greatly by researcher. For the purposes of this exercise, the emphasis was on the interview process rather than the collection of a full life history, and the interview time span was much less than for a full life history, which can involve many interviews, periods of participant observation, and collection of other data over months or even years.

Verification and Comment

Verification was first accomplished with the key informant. This is not always necessary, but sometimes tapes are unclear or the researcher might want to make sure he or she understood the point the person was making. It is a courtesy to do this and is strongly recommended. Next, the students communicated with the professor individually and then met as a group to share data and verify each other's analysis of the interviews. This involved a long meeting at which each student discussed the interviews thoroughly, exchanged notes, and argued about emergent themes. Once everyone felt comfortable with analysis, the final report could be written.

SUMMARY

Evaluation of the course by the students indicated that this exercise not only taught them a method that they had not considered but also provided a practical and supervised exercise in interviewing for research. The life histories collected for the course could easily be expanded into full life histories.

REFERENCES

de Chesnay, M. (2005). "Can't keep me down": Life histories of successful African American adults. In M. de Chesnay (Ed.), *Caring for the vulnerable*. Sudbury, MA: Jones & Bartlett.

de Chesnay, M., Rassilyer-Bomers, R., Webb, J., & Peil, R. (2008). Life histories of successful survivors of colostomy surgery, multiple sclerosis, and bereavement. In M. de Chesnay & B. Anderson (Eds.), *Caring for the vulnerable* (2nd ed.). Sudbury, MA: Jones & Bartlett.

de Chesnay, M., Walsh, L., Szekes, L., Kronawitter, V., Cox. K., Young, S., & Payne, H. (2012). In M. de Chesnay & B. Anderson (Eds.), *Caring for the vulnerable* (3rd ed.). Sudbury, MA: Jones & Bartlett.

CHAPTER TEN

LOSING A CHILD TO BRAINSTEM TUMOR: LIFE HISTORY OF NORA

Brenda Brown

INTERVIEW PROCESS FOR LIFE HISTORY

Description of Participant

The person I chose to interview was a woman in her 50s who had lost a grandchild to brain tumor. This woman is a nurse and a sister to one of the author's coworkers. When the child was ill, the coworker had discussed openly with others the initial diagnosis, the treatments, the progress, and finally the death of the child. Additionally, the woman and I had attended the same nursing program for a year about 30 years previously, though we had not maintained contact. For the purposes of this chapter, the participant will be referred to as Nora (all names are fictitious).

Nora is a nurse and works as the manager of surgical services at a large hospital system in the southeast. Her position puts her in close contact with numerous surgeons including neurosurgeons, so Nora is familiar with types of tumors and their treatment and outcomes. This knowledge was both a blessing and a burden as she faced the situation with her grandson. Nora looks very much like her sister who is the author's coworker. Their voices and laughs are quite similar. They both talk fast with a typical southern drawl and have an infectious hearty laugh. Yet, they can also be moved to tears quickly, especially when feeling compassion and empathy. Nora is the type of woman who would defend to the death anyone she cares about but could also let loose a tirade if she thinks someone deserves her wrath.

Nora's character was evident as she shared her story. She is the eldest of four siblings and has close relationships with all of her family—immediate and distant. She was reared by loving parents who also believed in discipline. Both maternal and paternal grandparents were significantly involved with

Nora and her siblings, and family gatherings for Sunday dinners and other events were a source of strength and comfort. Although Nora stated that she no longer attended church, her home life had also cultivated a strong belief in god and prayer, which served as a support for this experience. I noted family as a major concept in the typology constructed from the interview.

Nora was married in 1980 and had two children, Sue in 1982 and Karen in 1984. Sue was married in 2006 and her son, Tim, was born in 2008. Tim was diagnosed with a brain tumor in September 2010 and died in June 2011. Tim had a sister born in June 2010 and a brother born after his death in November 2011. Tim remained active until a few weeks before his death. He was aware that he would have a new brother and picked out his name. Those few months were bittersweet for the family, and Nora laughed and cried as she told her story. The brief time frame of the experience contributed to another major concept—urgency—that the author noted in constructing the interview typology.

During the interview, Nora related that she had not had the experience of losing a close family member at such a young age, and she felt fortunate and blessed. However, Nora had a sense that, at some point, the family would face such a tragedy, but she was not prepared for just how closely the tragedy would impact her life. Since the interview, Nora has experienced another loss. Her father died in June 2013. He was in his 80s and had some chronic health problems but had remained active until the past few months. He died peacefully at home surrounded by family.

CHOOSING A PARTICIPANT

The initial interview assignment was presented by a doctoral professor to the three students in a qualitative research course as an exercise in interviewing. I considered several individuals to interview, but they did not meet the criteria of the study. The participants needed to have experienced a life trauma, be an adult, not be a relative of the interviewer, and have successfully overcome the adversity. Finally, I invited a coworker who had cared for her terminally ill husband until he died several years ago. However, this coworker declined because she felt that she would not be able to revisit the experience.

I then considered another coworker's family and first asked about interviewing the mother of the child who died. This young woman would be a niece to the coworker. The coworker contacted her niece, who agreed to be interviewed but was unavailable at that time. When discussing the situation further with the coworker, I realized that the distance and schedule were not conducive to meeting in time to complete the assignment. So I then approached the coworker about interviewing her sister, the grandmother of the child. This woman agreed, and I was given contact information to set up a time and location for the interview. The connections of nursing school, working with the woman's sister, and having already heard the story were compelling reasons that I chose to interview this particular individual.

Once I had the contact information, I e-mailed the participant to introduce myself and to set up a mutually convenient time and location. The woman lived near my university, so we agreed to meet on an evening when I would be staying in the area and in a hotel room. The participant and I had communicated several times by e-mail and phone to verify time and location and to update on a few personal experiences since we had last seen each other.

Setting the Stage for the Interview

On the day I was to drive to the hotel, I had some errands to complete near home before starting the drive. After completing the last errand and returning to my car, I received a phone call from a friend in another state. The call was totally unexpected, so I was quite surprised. However, the friend was calling to inform me that a person close to me had just been talking to this friend and had expressed suicidal thoughts. The friend was quite concerned and felt that someone else should be aware of the situation. This friend had been unable to make contact with the person's mother. As soon as the conversation ended, I called the person who at that moment was in town and less than a mile away. We agreed to meet at my office very close by to discuss the next steps. After meeting and making some phone calls to family and facilities, the decision was made to take her to a psychiatric facility about 2 miles away for evaluation. Another family member was coming to stay with her so that I could leave in time to make the interview appointment. During the drive, the participant and I were in communication about the family emergency and the possibility of the meeting being delayed a few minutes. I arrived at the hotel and was able to get settled and order a delivery of pizza before the participant called to say she was in the lobby of the hotel.

I met the participant in the lobby and was happy to see the woman again after so many years. I remarked about how much the woman looked and sounded like her sister who is my coworker. On the walk to the hotel room, we shared some small talk and were comfortable with each other. When both of us were in the room and seated, I explained the purpose of the interview and the study. The consent form was reviewed and signed after the participant was given a chance to ask questions. She had none and signed three copies of the consent and was given one to keep (the other two being for the principal investigator [PI] and myself). Then the interview itself began.

The situation with the suicidal person had created a significant amount of concern and anxiety, and I wondered if I would be able to put the event aside to conduct the interview. Additionally, the interview process was a new experience, and I felt overwhelmed and ill-equipped to conduct the interview appropriately. However, I was able to put other concerns out of mind and concentrate on the interview. After the first couple of questions, I began to relax, and the interview continued for an hour and a half. The participant also seemed relaxed and was able to share her story. Occasionally, she had tears but was not embarrassed to cry. Overall, the interview experience was positive for both the author and the participant.

Two events that I had experienced made the subject matter of importance and interest. One was living in an abusive marriage. The resources I used to deal with the marriage and then the subsequent breakup of the marriage and divorce included spirituality, community organizations, and the support of family and friends. The second experience was that of surviving a tornado that hit my home in April 2011. This experience was different in that I did not expect to feel such emotional trauma from the event. The home was damaged, but no one was injured. Many others had suffered a great deal more loss from tornadoes during that season. Guilt for feeling traumatized was an overriding emotional result for me. As the home could be repaired and no one was injured or killed, I thought that I did not have the right to feel traumatized. Additionally, I felt abandoned by family and friends because only one coworker had come to visit during the summer break and only a few family members or friends had offered to help with the cleanup. I was unable to deal with this situation without the intervention of a health care professional. In fact, I had mentioned to classmates that I was willing to be interviewed as a survivor of trauma but upon reconsideration could not say I had dealt successfully with the experience or had recovered completely.

INTERVIEW RESULTS

Typology

The three main concepts from this interview seemed to be family, urgency, and coping. The subconcepts of family were the importance of, support from, and being with. Throughout the interview, Nora talked about family and came across as having a very strong sense of family relationship and a conviction of the "importance of family." For instance, she and her daughter, who lived a long distance away, talked on the phone nearly every day. Nora is also in close touch with her siblings and parents, as well as her extended family. She also spoke of her grandparents with respect and love. Nora related two stories she read when her grandson was still alive. Both stories involved parents who put their own needs or desires before those of their children, and Nora stated that those stories made her mad. "Support from family" during the illness and death of Nora's grandson was demonstrated in the way that immediate and extended family helped out with whatever was needed— transportation, food, supplies, and errands. "Being with family" was first displayed by the fact that Sue wanted her mother (Nora) to come immediately when she had received the news that Tim had a brain tumor. She said, "Mom, I need you to get out here." By contrast, Nora reported her son-in-law's family as being loving but used to being apart because of the military. Jim's parents did not have the finances to fly out to be with them when the diagnosis was first made. But Nora said she was going whether she had the money or not. While Nora's grandson was undergoing treatment and during the last days, being with family was one thing in which they all found comfort. Nora mentioned a couple of times that being with her grandson and granddaughter was a way of coping. Another way in which the importance of family was demonstrated was when Jim's grandmother wanted Tim to be baptized even though Sue and Jim did not feel he needed to be. But Sue's feeling was that if baptizing Tim would give the grandmother peace, then it was okay.

A sense of urgency was another concept that seemed to dominate the interview with Nora. The first subconcept appeared to be the urgency to know the truth. When Sue noticed the crossed eye in her son, she immediately notified a physician who examined him. She was then directed to take her son right away to a major medical center for further testing. From the hospital in the southwest, Sue, Nora, and the children went immediately to the children's hospital in the southeast. Both Nora and her husband (Don) flew to be with Sue and Jim right away. Because the hospital in the SW was an hour from Sue and Jim's home, they did not return to the home to pack up any belongings. Don and Jim took Sue, Nora, and the children to an airport so that they could get to the children's hospital as soon as possible. Don and Jim drove 18 hours straight through. The following day, the oncologist met with the family to give them the news that the brain tumor was quite aggressive and that Tim had 9 months at best. At no time did Nora mention any desire from Sue and Jim or her and Don to delay knowing the diagnosis and starting treatment. The second subconcept was the urgency to enjoy what was left—meaning the time that Tim had left. Sue and Jim were determined to make Tim's last months as pleasant as possible. They did not want anyone crying in front of him. The family took two trips to a theme park, so Tim could have some fun. Even near the end of Tim's life, the family—including the extended family—stayed together in Sue and Jim's home, so they could be close and make the most of every moment they had.

The third concept—coping—has several subconcepts. Nora mentioned that she and Sue were just "doing the best they could." The treatment decisions and day-to-day care of Tim also communicated that Sue and Jim and the rest of the family were trying to do their best. I believe this "doing their best" gave them comfort in dealing with a completely unexpected and tragic situation. The second subconcept was "accepting help or care." Friends, family, coworkers, and strangers helped in many ways, and their help was never turned down. Nora noted in the interview the number of people "coming out of the woodwork" to help and she—as well as Don, Sue, and Jim—were very grateful for the support. Nora mentioned the hospice nurse—a lady in her 80s—and how much support she was during the last weeks.

Another major source of help was a man in Jim's unit who volunteered to go to Afghanistan in his place. The military was helpful in finding a position for Jim, so he could be close to his wife and children. "Spirituality and faith" were strong coping mechanisms. Nora's grandparents were instrumental in her development of spiritual beliefs by living a life of faith. Nora shared that she never blamed or was angry with god, and that she believed she would see Tim again. She appreciated the ministers who came to offer comfort. "Having a routine" was another coping mechanism. During radiation and chemotherapy, Tim did not suffer much from side effects, so Nora could play with him as usual. After those therapies were completed, maintaining normalcy as much as possible made the situation manageable. Nora said that being with Tim helped her forget he was terminally ill. Finally, "telling their story" has brought much comfort to Sue and Nora. They have raised money for childhood brain tumor research. Sue has shared her story at fundraisers, with nursing students, and on the Internet. She and Nora have plans to write a book about Tim. Nora said that people were hesitant to mention Tim, but she has told them she wants to talk about him and share his story. Nora believes that going on with life—and not giving up—is what honors Tim.

DISCUSSION

Traumatic life events call forth various coping methods determined by many factors. An individual's age, specific event, culture, gender, family values, support system, and religious beliefs are a few of those factors. People often propose how they would cope with a given situation, but until that event happens they cannot know for certain. What seems to matter most in coping with traumatic life events is that the individual must decide what is and is not helpful. Some behaviors in one culture would be considered bizarre in another. Societal norms also impact the manner in which people cope. In the United States, a person suffering the loss of a close relative is usually granted 3 days for bereavement. Yet, how can an employer decide that 3 days are enough? People who lose beloved pets are not granted any time off for bereavement, and again, who has the right to decide that losing a pet is not as great a loss? Does keeping that "stiff upper lip" in the face of tragedy make someone a better person?

A literature search using the words "coping with traumatic event" and filtered for the years 2007 to 2013, scholarly journals, and full text yielded 43,981 hits. The literature included studies that focused on gender, age, nationality, specific events, religiosity, professions, and numerous other factors and the methods, abilities, and physiological responses of the brain in coping with trauma. Thus, this topic has been well studied by many researchers and practitioners for decades.

Bonanno, Pat-Horenczyk, and Noll (2011) discussed the development of a scale to measure the ability to deal with traumatic events. The researchers had completed an extensive review of literature related to coping with trauma. An individual's ability to cope with trauma is not limited to one method. As coping is such a personal and individualized concept, perhaps it is best considered in the context of the factors mentioned in the preceding paragraph. Certainly some coping methods are healthier than others. For instance, murdering the drunk driver who caused the accident that killed a child might seem reasonable to the parent at the time. However, the outcome for the parent would most likely result in a worse situation such as a prison sentence. Some individuals develop a personality disorder related to sexual abuse as a child. Given the emotional liability and other characteristics of that disorder, it does not seem a healthy method for long-term coping. Yet one can understand a child's immediate need to deal with the situation.

One personal experience of mine led to coping methods that were not healthy. In the case of living with an abusive spouse, the coping method for a long time was denial and self-blaming. However, eventually, those methods resulted in significant physical pain, suicidal ideation, and anorexia. When I made the decision to seek professional help, I learned healthier coping skills that empowered me to change and leave the situation. Thus, coping methods are not necessarily right or wrong but can result in unhealthy behaviors, thoughts, and emotions that bring about a worse state for the individual than before the traumatic event.

SUMMARY OF WHAT I LEARNED

My learning can be divided into two aspects—personal coping and qualitative interviewing. The personal coping aspect is based on the experience of the tornado. The morning following the tornado, when the damage was visible, the overwhelming feeling was shock. The home and property appeared to have been hit by a bomb. The priority was to remove trees, so the driveway would be cleared. Several days later, the author was able to let go of pent up emotion and cry. However, shortly after, guilt became a pervasive emotion because, in my case, no life had been lost and comparatively little damage had been done to the home. Many people had died, lost loved ones, or lost entire homes and personal belongings in that same tornado. I felt that my situation was not as severe as others, so why would I deserve empathy. I had read about survivor guilt but had not experienced this emotion until this event.

During the summer following the tornado, I began to experience a great deal of anxiety and depression and was afraid to be alone. Additionally, several severe storms had hit the area again, and each time, I relived the experience of the tornado. Loud sudden noises were especially disturbing and frightening. The house was being repaired, so workers were coming and going, along with insurance agents and others. My privacy was invaded, and I rarely had quiet time. The depression and anxiety continued to increase, as well as frequent bouts of crying. Eventually a coworker noticed and emphasized the need to seek professional help. I was able to recognize that I suffered from post-traumatic stress disorder (PTSD).

More than 2 years have passed since the tornado, and I feel that only just now have I recovered from the trauma. The intensity of emotions, the length of recovery, and the need for professional care were not what I expected to experience. In fact, that fall semester, I began a doctoral program and because of the PTSD was almost unable to complete the coursework. I have become more empathetic and understanding of PTSD and of how long a traumatic event may affect an individual.

The second aspect was learning the interview process. Finding someone to interview and asking to interview that person about a traumatic event were more difficult than I expected. The interview is invasive no matter how professionally and empathetically it is done. The researcher must have and display the utmost respect for the participant.

Conducting the interview was not a comfortable experience for me. Even though the participant and I were open, friendly, and respectful and I asked the right questions, practicing active listening takes skill. When I began the interview, the thought flashed through my mind "You are in way over your head." Role playing may be a way to lessen this discomfort and anxiety about conducting real research interviews.

Finally, the hours before conducting an interview should be free of stressful situations as much as possible. The situation with the suicidal person and having to drive a distance in heavy traffic to meet the appointment time added to the anxiety. Probably the better thing would have been to reschedule the interview, but my time constraints were not conducive to rescheduling. However, the opportunity to conduct a study interview was valuable and can be a building block for future opportunities.

REFERENCE

Bonanno, G., Pat-Horenczyk, R., & Noll, J. (2011). Coping flexibility and trauma: The perceived ability to cope with trauma (PACT) scale. *Psychological Trauma: Theory, Research, Practice, and Policy, 3*(2), 117–129. doi:10.1037/a0020921

CHAPTER ELEVEN

SUCCESSFULLY OVERCOMING
BREAST CANCER: NICOLE'S STORY

Katrina Embrey

This life history was completed as a doctoral course requirement for qualitative methods. I chose to interview Nicole because I thought she would be an ideal candidate to meet the goals of the qualitative interview assignment, which was to conduct a life history on someone who had successfully overcome adversity.

THE PARTICIPANT

Nicole (pseudonym) is a 26-year-old Caucasian female who is completing her junior year in a baccalaureate nursing program. Nicole was born and raised in a mid-sized city in the Southeastern United States. Religion was an integral part of her cultural background while growing up, as she and her family attended church regularly. She was baptized at age 11. She is the oldest of three children and is from a middle-class family. She has two siblings— one younger sister and one younger brother. Her parents divorced when she was a teenager, and she lived with her father until the age of 18. She then moved in with her boyfriend and became pregnant with her son, who is now 5 years old, and subsequently got married. At age 22, she discovered a nonhealing sore on her breast. After a prolonged period of misdiagnoses by a gynecologist, breast surgeon, and dermatologist, she was finally diagnosed with Padgett's disease and breast cancer at age 24, after seeing a second breast surgeon. She received a mastectomy and chemotherapy as treatment. She currently lives with her husband and young son and is enrolled as a full-time nursing student. Nicole has been cancer-free for 2 years and 4 months.

I had considered interviewing two other women who had lived through the experiences of breast cancer and ovarian cancer but, after careful consideration, decided on Nicole for two reasons. First, each of the other two women were related to me, and therefore I, as the interviewer, was too close to the subjects and could not be far enough removed from their experiences to conduct a successful interview. Second, the woman who had ovarian cancer was in the midst of treatment, and it was not known that she had successfully overcome this adversity at that time. I decided on Nicole as my interviewee because she had identified herself as a "survivor" of breast cancer and was successfully progressing in the baccalaureate nursing program of study. Not only was she a survivor but also she was unique in the fact that she had developed breast cancer at such a young age. I thought it would be interesting to explore the perspective on adversity of someone who was in his or her early twenties. I felt she qualified as having overcome this adversity because she had been cancer-free for over 2 years at the time of the interview and she was an active participant in her life.

THE INTERVIEW PROCESS

Once the decision on whom to interview was made, the process began with recruitment. Nicole had been made known to me by a faculty member in the nursing school that Nicole attended. The faculty member had been one of Nicole's clinical instructors, and during a physical assessment lab assignment, Nicole verbalized her ordeal with breast cancer and how she now wanted to help others. I first approached Nicole via e-mail and told her about the study and asked if she would be willing to talk to me. She responded and gave me her phone number, and I called her. We spoke on the phone, and I gave a more detailed explanation of the study and that it would require an in-depth personal interview that would last no longer than 1 to 1½ hours. I told her that, after the first interview, subsequent interviews of shorter duration might be needed to clarify responses. Nicole agreed to meet me and participate in the study. We set up a time to meet that was convenient for her. The location was of her choice, and she preferred to meet in an office on a college campus.

Nicole and I met at the agreed on time. To begin the interview process, I thanked her for her willingness to participate and explained the study. I explained that her identity would remain anonymous, and she had the opportunity to choose a pseudonym. She chose "Nicole." Informed consent was obtained prior to beginning the interview. The written consent was reviewed and Nicole had a chance to read the form and was given the opportunity to ask any questions. Upon approval of the form, Nicole signed two copies, one of which was given to her and the researcher kept the other.

I obtained permission from Nicole to tape the interview, asked if she was comfortable and if she needed anything such as water, and then began the interview process. I began the interview using a template of seven questions and format for genogram and timeline as provided by de Chesnay and colleagues (2012). To protect Nicole's privacy, the answers to these are not included in this chapter. The interview process progressed easily because Nicole talked freely and extensively in response to each of the questions. Nicole answered the initial questions in a very matter of fact way until the first question about her feelings was asked. At this time, her mood changed and she became contemplative. I found it difficult to deal with the silence at times but remembered that Dr. de Chesnay had said that if an interviewer will wait and accept the silence that is so awkward, the person being interviewed will reveal important information. During these moments of silence, I found it hard to not interject my own thoughts of the situation.

Once the interview questions turned toward Nicole's feelings and family, she became emotional to the point of tears. I offered her tissues and encouraged her as she spoke. She continued the interview despite the crying. When the questions changed from a focus on her feelings to a focus on her support and coping mechanisms, she stopped crying with the exception of an occasional tear. At the conclusion of the questions, I asked Nicole for family information that would allow me to complete a genogram. I ended the interview by thanking her for her time and told her that I would contact her again if needed. Overall, the interview process went well. I was nervous at first, as I did not know what would happen or how successful I would be as an interviewer. Difficulties came with the periods of silence. It was hard to know how long to sit in silence and whether to prompt her to continue. It was also emotional at times for the interviewer. Listening to Nicole's story and seeing the wide range of emotions the questions elicited was sobering. I also found myself crying as she relieved the moments of pain and joy as she told her story.

THE ANALYSIS

The most challenging part of conducting the life history was the analysis of the data. The writing of the transcript was very time consuming, as each word had to be transcribed exactly as it was verbalized. It was hard to write the spoken word. After the interview was transcribed, the transcript was read in its entirety. During the second reading of the content and the process, concepts began to emerge. Several more readings were conducted until the main concepts were identified. A draft of the data was shared with two other doctoral students who each reviewed the data. The concepts were discussed and agreed on and were organized using a typology chart.

RESULTS

Four main concepts emerged from the data analysis for this interview: coping, caring, finding meaning, and emotional processing. The first main concept was coping. Coping is defined as the "way" in which Nicole was able to overcome the many difficulties that she experienced throughout the breast cancer treatment. The methods Nicole used to cope were identified as subconcepts and included family support, spirituality, and telling her story. Family support was found predominately in three male members of her family, her husband, father, and son. Although she had a mother, sister, and brother, she stated she did not find support from any family members other than her husband, father, and son. She had never had a very close relationship with her mother in the past, and this time was no exception. Her siblings seemed to remain distant throughout the experience. Her father and husband provided support by "being there" and listening when she needed to talk. Having her son in her life was a factor in motivating her to appear strong, as she did not want her son to always see her crying. The second subconcept of coping was spirituality. Spirituality is defined as having faith and praying to the Lord. Nicole prayed to the Lord when she felt fearful or when she could not talk to her husband or father. She made the comment, "I just prayed, and you know, that's all I could do." Prayer was used to talk to the Lord, and getting her feelings out in this way made her feel better and confident that everything would eventually get better. Prayer gave her strength, which she said she needed to deal with "it." The third subconcept of coping was "telling her story." Nicole was very eager to tell her story and has shared her experience with others. She felt that making others aware of her situation has helped her and she would continue to tell her story as often as she is asked. This subconcept of telling her story closely relates to two other main concepts that were identified as caring and finding meaning.

The second main concept was caring. The type of caring that was evident in the data was caring for others, especially her son, father, and husband. Nicole often made comments about her concern for her husband's and father's feelings and how she did not want to burden them, worry them, or make them sad. She made comments about the possibility of not being there for her son and how her son needs a "mommy." She wants more children but has a conflict because she is concerned for the unborn children because of the possibility of giving them a first-generation relative with breast cancer. She did not want her son to see her crying all the time or appearing "sickly." Nicole showed concern for strangers in a supermarket. She commented that she was probably rude to them on the day she found out she had cancer and was concerned that she did not smile at them that day or that she was rude. She made a comment that the experience had made her think of others and consider their unique situation prior to judging their actions. She realizes now that one never knows what another person is going through until one has walked in his or her shoes. When asked if she was afraid to die, her answer was no, not because of herself but yes, because she would be concerned about leaving her son without a mother.

The third main concept was "finding meaning." Finding meaning is defined as a way of making sense of the adversity. Early in the diagnosis, Nicole asked why it was happening to her, but once she started chemotherapy, she changed to believing there was a reason for it happening. The reason it happened was so that she would help others and make a difference in their lives. She made a statement, "I just think this whole cancer diagnosis was for a reason . . . I think maybe it was to make me a better person and a better nurse." "Everything that happened to me had a purpose, was for a reason."

The fourth main concept was "emotional processing." Throughout the interview, there were many emotions expressed such as anger, sadness, pain, fear, and relief. Each of the negative emotions were "processed" in some way and resulted in a positive feeling. For example, "breast cancer was everybody's fear, but I was like almost relieved because I know what it was, that it can be fixed." She commented that when she was scared, she would tell herself that after "getting it all out," it would give her a sense of relief. The anger she felt toward her original medical team that misdiagnosed her and made her feel so unimportant has been balanced by the positive feelings for the new medical team that has helped her feel important. When asked to find one word or phrase to describe how she knew she had overcome this adversity, she said, "I almost feel maybe a sense of relief that the worst is behind me."

DISCUSSION

The decision to study Nicole's life, an atypical case of breast cancer, began as an exercise in conducting the steps in the process of a life history methodology. The process of conducting this life history increased my awareness of the profound effect this qualitative research methodology can have on individuals. In the end, it was much more than a learning exercise in qualitative research; it was an example of healing. McElligott (2010) gives an operational definition of healing as "the personal experience of transcending suffering and transforming to wholeness, resulting in serenity, interconnectedness, and a new sense of meaning" (p. 258). Nicole's story and the process of telling her story through nursing research can be viewed as facilitating healing. Not only has Nicole been physically healed from cancer, but she has also transcended the suffering of the experience and has developed a new sense of meaning in her life. She has found meaning in the experience to become a better person and a more compassionate nurse. Nicole's healing process continued through the interview process. She wants to tell her story, and telling her story makes her feel better. This is evident in her quote, "I don't mind telling my story and letting anybody know what happened to me because if one person hears what happened to me and it makes them go have a mammogram or do their breast self-exam and if it saves somebody's life, then everything that I went through was worth it." That statement is a powerful example of how conducting qualitative nursing research in life histories can have a positive effect on those who have overcome adversity as well as others who hear their stories.

REFERENCES

de Chesnay, M., Walsh, L., Szekes, L., Kronawitter, V., Cox. K., Young, S., & Payne, H. (2012). In M. de Chesnay & B. Anderson (Eds.), *Caring for the vulnerable* (3rd ed.). Sudbury, MA: Jones & Bartlett.

McElligott, D. (2010). Healing: The journey from concept to nursing practice. *Journal of Holistic Nursing, 28,* 251–259.

CHAPTER TWELVE

OVERCOMING SUBSTANCE ABUSE: LIFE HISTORY OF ALEXA

Nancy Capponi

The process of interviewing a study participant, transcribing the interview, and analyzing the narrative transcript is both challenging and rewarding. The rewards of the process are worth the researcher's efforts. Narrative analysis provides insight into another person's perspective regarding the meanings that life events hold for that person. In this particular case, the interpretive approach of a life history supplied rich data about a specific life-changing or epiphanal event in a person's life (Denszin & Lincoln, 2005).

DESCRIPTION OF THE PERSON

At the time of the interview for the life history, the interviewee was a 36-year-old college student in the last semester of a baccalaureate program. I had known Alexa for about a year when the interview occurred. She was a senior collegiate student who was conscientious in her studies. Alexa maintained a high grade-point average and was inducted into the honor society during her last semester of university.

Alexa is mature, knowledgeable, likeable, and sure of herself, without any hints of a difficult past. She is Caucasian, with a German Welsh ethnicity and a middle-class socioeconomic status. The interviewee has never been married and has a Presbyterian religious affiliation. Her family includes her divorced parents and an older brother, all within easy driving distance. She is well-liked by her peers, and she boasts of a large group of supportive friends and acquaintances.

I was acquainted with Alexa, the student, having been one of her faculty for two semesters. I was unaware of the struggles she had had to undergo to get to this point in her life until another student, in the course of a conversation about drug abuse, brought it to my attention. When an assignment to interview someone who had overcome adversity to achieve life goals needed to be completed for one of my doctoral courses, I thought of Alexa. The brief information I received about her intrigued me, and I wanted to learn more about this person and how she had achieved her current status.

The interviewee overcame the adversity of alcohol and drug abuse to successfully graduate from a baccalaureate college program, with solid support from friends and family. Alexa has strong convictions and, by her account, has to "work" her program of recovery every day. She states that some days are easier than others, but, generally, it has gotten easier over time. When observing Alexa and her interactions with others, it was difficult for me to imagine this wonderful, caring person as an alcohol and drug abuser with a dysfunctional life.

DESCRIPTION OF RECRUITMENT AND INTERVIEW

Recruitment

I initially approached Alexa in a private place on campus and informed her how I had learned about her overcoming an adversity to get to her current successful circumstances. I described the course assignment first. I then recounted the reasons that I believed she would be an excellent interviewee for this assignment. I did disclose how I had learned about her history. I reviewed the interview process including the fact that there would probably be more than one interview involved as well as follow-up telephone and/or e-mail discussions. The use of her life history as part of a future textbook on life histories edited by my instructor was also discussed. Voluntary participation in the interview was stressed, and I communicated that refusal to collaborate in the process would have no negative consequences to the interviewee. I assured her more than once that her anonymity as the interviewee would be maintained and that a detailed consent form outlining all aspects of the interview process would need to be signed before any aspect of the collaboration began. Alexa readily agreed to participate in the assignment.

Interview Process

Initial Interview

The initial interview with the participant took place at a place and time mutually agreed on. Alexa chose to meet in a meeting room in a large building on campus that was convenient for her and where she felt comfortable.

Privacy was ensured by locking the door, and all communication devices were turned off except for the digital recorder.

The meeting room was quiet and private without any distractions. The second, lengthy interview occurred in the same meeting room on campus, again with all communication devices turned off. Short discussions and question–answer sessions occurred by e-mail and telephone conversations over the course of 6 weeks. A digital recorder was utilized during the two face-to-face interviews, and a brief note-taking was undertaken by the interviewer. The participant was reminded that the interviews were being recorded and assured that the recordings would be kept for a period of 3 years in a secure place and then erased.

To maintain anonymity, an alias for the participant was created for the transcription and analysis of the interview. The name, Alexa, was chosen by the participant and no explanation of her choice was ever revealed. All other persons mentioned in Alexa's life history were assigned aliases by the interviewer (with approval from Alexa) to maintain the anonymity of the participant.

During the initial interview, I reviewed the informed consent document (approval had been obtained earlier for this study) with the interviewee. The interviewee expressed no objections, concerns, or questions regarding the interview. The informed consent was signed by the participant voluntarily. I emphasized that the consent could be revoked at any time during the interview process without recriminations and stressed the voluntary nature of this project. I encouraged the interviewee to ask questions throughout the process.

Maintaining a relaxed environment was important for the interview to progress. I provided the refreshments required or requested by Alexa. Background noise was minimal or nonexistent, consisting of nature noises (birds) outside the meeting room windows. The room chosen was large and had a locked door, and it had comfortable chairs and a table. Interruptions to the interview were unlikely in the meeting room (and did not occur). The lighting in the room was bright enough to take notes but not too bright. The digital recorder was unobtrusive.

The initial interview was shortened to thirty minutes because of the fact that Alexa had worked the previous night and had forgotten the pictures that she wanted to use during the interview. The informed consent provided by the course instructor was reviewed and signed with the interviewee, the interviewer receiving a copy and the original returned to the course instructor. Basic demographic and background information was obtained during the first encounter.

The second, lengthy interview occurred a week later in a similar location. This interview lasted an hour and a half without a break. I took brief notes but for the most part maintained a good eye contact with Alexa and allowed her to tell her story. The interview was semi-structured in that several questions within the assignment were included. Alexa was encouraged to tell her life history in her own words and manner, making the interview mostly unstructured. Alexa used pictures to identify family and friends and to relate incidents and situations each of them was involved in, during her narration. She was verbose and had little difficulty in recounting the events of her life. As illustrated in the interview transcript, Alexa answered all my questions in a frank and honest manner and openly discussed her life history with me.

Challenges

The interview process was not without its challenges. Choosing the interviewee could have been problematic. I was fortunate to have found out about the participant because I knew of only one other person who had overcome adversity to achieve career success; however, I felt that this person still had lingering emotional issues regarding the adverse event and did not feel particularly inspired to interview her. Alexa was a good choice for me; her life history fit the interview guidelines, and she met the sample inclusion criteria of the assignment. She amazed me with her outlook and what she had already achieved in her life despite or because of her continuing battle with alcohol and substance abuse.

The actual interview itself was not difficult to accomplish. I had a cooperative and talkative interviewee who did not hesitate to share her feelings and emotions as well as the events of her life. There were moments when I became emotional about situations that had happened to Alexa and, when she completed her narrative, I felt proud of her and her accomplishments. Several follow-up e-mails and brief telephone calls after the initial and second interview occurred during the next month for clarification of details and to answer other questons that arose. Alexa was patient and cooperative throughout the process.

Transcribing the interviews took several hours because I was striving for accuracy. Some of the nonverbal communication may have been missed, as I was concentrating on listening attentively to Alexa as she spoke. Alexa maintained a stoic or flat facial affect for most of her narrative, but did show some emotion, with tears and hesitation in her speech at some points of her story. The interview transcript analysis consisted of the following: the actual interview content or raw word-for-word data along with descriptions of the interviewer observations; significant reactions of Alexa or the interviewer during the interview; statements regarding the context of the data, and clarification/making sense of the situations and emotions involved; and concepts and themes that emerged from the data. The process took several hours and much thought. Throughout the interview, I had no ethnocentric bias that I was aware of. During our interviews and later conversations, Alexa repeatedly stated that the actions she had taken during her recovery process were *her* choices and might not necessarily work for others in a similar situation.

RESULTS

The genogram (not included for reasons of privacy) for Alexa reveals family relationships and some of the medical and social issues among them. Alexa attempted to get information on her aunts and uncles from both of her parents and did state that there may be some missing information on the health histories. Alexa's parents, aunts, and uncles are middle-aged to older adults, with all but one maternal grandmother deceased. Her cousins are close to Alexa's age or slightly older.

In Alexa's parents' generation, between the two families, five aunts/ uncles are currently married (one paternal uncle is in his second marriage), with one current divorce (her parents), three maternal aunts who have never married, one paternal aunt who died as an adult, and one maternal aunt who died as an infant. Two of Alexa's father's siblings were diagnosed with cancer (sister died and brother had prostate cancer), and one of Alexa's mother's siblings (brother) had basal cell carcinoma. Both families (paternal sister, maternal sister) have incidences of hypertension. Two of Alexa's maternal aunts also have hypothyroidism. Alexa was unable to get a medical history from one of her paternal uncles. Of note is the fact that both Alexa's parents have a history of depression and high cholesterol. Alexa states that her mother is very "codependent," and throughout her life, she has focused on taking care of others first. Both Alexa's father and brother have battled with substance abuse: her father with alcohol and her older brother with drug abuse as a teenager.

In addition, the timeline of Alexa's life demonstrates significant events from her birth to the time of the interview. Alexa's mother's near-fatal motor vehicle accident when Alexa was 7 years old was the first event that Alexa recalls having affected her emotionally. Apparently, it took months for her mother to recover and required the assistance of one of her maternal aunts. Alexa states that she did not understand what was wrong with her mother and that she constantly feared that her mother would die.

Alexa's father had a history of depression, and when Alexa was 10 years old, he attempted suicide. A year later, her parents divorced. Not only does Alexa recall how sad she was at the time but how much she missed her father and the family life she had previously loved. She also felt that perhaps if she had been a better daughter, the divorce might not have happened.

Throughout her adolescent years, starting at age 14, Alexa tried alcohol and marijuana, experimented with lysergic acid diethylamide (LSD) and cocaine, and abused her methylphenidate (Ritalin) prescription. At age 16, Alexa became so depressed that she attempted suicide with pills. Alexa became more depressed the following year when a male friend of hers committed suicide. Her high school grades, previously straight A's, began to plummet until, in 1994, she dropped out of high school. Alexa did obtain her graduate education diploma (GED) when she was 20 years old and then made two unsuccessful attempts at starting college, which ended in poor grades and her dropping out.

Alexa's substance abuse lasted for more than 10 years. She states that there were a lot of "ups and downs" during this period (1993–2004), with times when her life felt good. As time went on, however, Alexa says that she became less productive as a member of society, more depressed, and more alienated from her family and friends. In her early to mid-20s, at the height of her substance abuse, Alexa was asked to leave her father's house, failed to keep her well-paying job, lost her car (was impounded), had another friend commit suicide, and got into trouble with the law, eventually ending up in jail more than one time.

In her late 20s, Alexa began her recovery from alcohol/drug abuse with a rehabilitation program that worked and continues to work for her. She states that she had a relapse in 2007 when another friend died (causes unknown). Alexa has had a stable home environment and supportive family and friends throughout her recovery and has gradually allowed those close to her to be a part of her life again.

In the year that this interview was completed, 36-year-old Alexa became a college graduate and is currently happily pursuing her chosen career. Alexa is a well-liked person who struggles to maintain her sobriety and life without drugs. During rehabilitation, Alexa states that she set up rules for herself and follows them strictly. She says that this is the only way for her to maintain control of her life and to avoid situations that are not healthy for her.

Clearly delineated are the years and events discussed in the interview that led to Alexa's overcoming alcohol addiction and drug abuse to become a successful person with achievable life goals and objectives. She is a strong, motivated person who seems happy with her current life course.

ANALYSIS

The analysis of the interview transcript included concepts and themes that emerged from the raw data. The use of a typology chart was essential to the organization of the concepts deduced from Alexa's interview. Each of the main concepts that emerged appears to be of high importance to Alexa and is exemplified in her narratives and responses to questions during the interview process.

The three main concepts found in the interview analysis are family/friends, caring, and coping. I included Alexa's friends as part of her extended family because all seem to be integral parts of much of her life and motivators for some of her actions during her addiction and in her rehabilitation. Examples of each concept and subconcept can be found throughout the interview.

The main theme of family/friends includes the subconcepts of the importance of family/friends, support from family/friends, the importance of being with family/friends, and a realistic view of family/friends' weaknesses, issues, and acceptance of these issues. The importance of family/friends is demonstrated in the interview transcripts—Alexa's obvious fear and sadness regarding her mother's near-fatal automobile accident and long convalescence; her father's job transfer, which kept him away from the family on weekdays for over a year; the loss of her family unit as a result of the divorce; the family atmosphere provided to her by a friend's family and her rehabilitation facility staff; disappointment and depression over a missed family Christmas during her addiction time; finding a new home with a friend's mother after the rehabilitation facility; and support from a church group over the years. The significance of Alexa's family/friends seems to have always been important to her and continues to be so today.

Support from family/friends is significant to Alexa, as she was given support by many people throughout her life. She sought out support from many people and lacked support from family/friends at times in her life, and, in a misguided attempt to protect her family/friends from herself during her addiction years, she detached or separated herself from everyone she cared about or who cared about her. There are other examples of support from family in the interview transcript such as support from friends' families as a teenager and an adult and meeting a friend's mother who took her into her home during Alexa's early rehabilitation years. She feels that the lack of support from her parents contributed to her depression and years of addiction.

Alexa expresses her devotion to her immediate family and friends; the importance of having people around her whom she can count on is found throughout the interview. She now counts on family/friends to provide support and returns that support when needed, as shown when her mother recently had financial issues and when a friend in recovery described her difficulty in her marriage because her husband smokes marijuana, and Alexa assisted them. Alexa does demonstrate a realistic view of her family/friends and acceptance of their weaknesses and issues. When talking about friends who have died, Alexa is emotional and saddened. She is equally proud of friends who are in recovery and is supportive of them.

The second main concept of caring is composed of the subconcepts of fear of hurting family/friends, codependency, fear of disappointing her family, control, care and concern for others (selflessness), embarrassment and shame, and depression. The concept of caring was apparent during the interview, from the emotions exhibited by Alexa and from her verbal/nonverbal expressions.

To me, the most poignant part of the interview was when Alexa described how she removed herself from her family's and friends' lives and distanced herself from everyone who cared about her. She stated that weeks or months would go by without her communicating with her family and letting her family be involved in her life. Alexa pretended her family was not there and described herself as a ghost who avoided family/friends during her years of heavy addiction. Alexa did not express during the interview her motives in separating herself from her family, so I can only infer that perhaps Alexa was either ashamed of what she was doing, afraid of disappointing or hurting her family, or wanted to protect her family/friends from the person she was during her addiction years. Alexa is currently a confident young woman who follows the rules, speaks honestly about herself, and has direction and purpose in her life with the support of her family/friends.

Depression is a subconcept that Alexa mentions at various times throughout the interview. She did attempt suicide as a teenager, and both her parents had also attempted suicide. Alexa mentions friends who attempted to, and who did, commit suicide.

Codependency is found in the interview in Alexa's perspective of her mother being codependent throughout her life. From my point of view, Alexa is also codependent. She genuinely cares for her family and friends and, I believe, sometimes unintentionally takes over and directs them, with good intentions. Alexa believes that control in her childhood home was gone when her father moved out and that she did lose control of her life during her addiction years. Alexa does have her rules and standards and follows each as a method of keeping her recovery intact and not relapsing.

The last theme of coping consists of the subconcepts of doing her best during difficult times, rationalization, accepting help and care from others, spirituality and faith, the importance of having a routine and of having rules, being emotionless during her narrations, and self-preservation. Alexa describes instances when she managed to get through difficult times to the best of her ability, such as when her mother was in a serious motor vehicle accident, her teenaged years and eventually dropping out of high school with a poor grade point average, the chaos of drug addiction, and the attempts at avoiding codependency by using drugs.

The subconcept of rationalization is seen when Alexa explains away her behaviors regarding her lack of sleep and her lifestyle to her high school friends. She rationalizes her mother's previous and current behaviors, such as her codependency in Alexa's childhood and her current financial dependence on Alexa. Rationalization is observed when Alexa describes stealing from a man who was seeking a prostitute and feeling that this is okay because he put himself in that situation. Alexa rationalizes many of her life choices including her addictions.

Spirituality and faith are interwoven throughout Alexa's life history. Alexa states that she never completely lost her faith even when she was deeply into her addictions, but she did put faith in the back of her mind and stop seeking it. When Alexa was at her lowest point (in jail), she did call on her faith to help her get out of her legal and addiction situations and to give her peace. Spirituality and faith are integral components of Alexa's life today.

Emotionlessness is a coping mechanism that Alexa employed during many parts of the interview. Throughout a lot of the interview, she maintained a flat affect with nearly a monotone voice. Self-preservation is another concept that is evident in the interview. Alexa is realistic and aware of potential triggers that may jeopardize her recovery and analyzes changes in her life carefully before making decisions about anything.

The significance of Alexa's family/friends seems to have always been extremely important to her and continues to be so today. Alexa demonstrates fear and sadness regarding many events in her life that involved either her family or friends including her mom's near-fatal automobile accident, the loss of her family unit to divorce, and the disappointment of missing Christmas with her family during her addiction. Alexa recognizes the significance of the support she received throughout her life from her family, friends, and acquaintances during her addiction years and in recovery.

The concept of caring is apparent from the emotions exhibited by Alexa and her verbal/nonverbal expressions during the interviews and conversations. One of the most poignant parts of the interview was when Alexa described how she removed herself from her family's and friends' lives and distanced herself from anyone who cared for her during her years of heavy addiction. She did not allow anyone who cared about her or whom she cared about to be involved in her life and even pretended that these people did not exist. Alexa was unclear about her motivations for this separation from family/friends during her addiction years but related the noncommunication during these years on her part. Some possibilities for this separation included embarrassment or shame, fear of disappointing or hurting her family/friends, and protecting her family/friends from the person she was during this period. The Alexa of today is a different person in many ways from the addict Alexa of the past: She is a thoughtful, confident young woman who follows the rules, speaks honestly about herself and her family/friends, and has direction and purpose in her life.

Alexa currently lives her life as a recovering addict. The concept of coping and how Alexa coped during different periods of her life are captured throughout the interview. The method of coping is developed by a person when a threat, event, or stressor is identified and evaluated by that individual. Adaptation to the situation is the result of successful coping (McEwen & Wills, 2011). During her addiction years, Alexa depended on no one but herself to get through the chaos of addiction. When events led Alexa to the point where she realized that nothing she was doing for herself was helping her life situation, and that her situation was only worsening, she finally accepted help from others. The Alexa recovering from addiction is realistic about potential triggers that may jeopardize her recovery and has a high level of self-preservation. Alexa relies on her family/friends, faith, and self-developed rules and routines to propel her through life.

WHAT I LEARNED FROM THIS EXPERIENCE

The process of planning and implementing a life history interview can be lengthy and requires skills developed by practice. As an experienced nurse, I have learned over time how to obtain a history from a patient or client. Purposeful, quality interviewing abilities are learned and improved by exposure to the process. It is difficult to understand another person's perspective even if the interviewer has been through something similar. Establishing rapport with the interviewee is crucial to the interview process.

The interview with Alexa was easy in that we were familiar with each other before the interview; however, it was difficult because of the new roles we had to fill for the interview. I found it difficult to ask questions in a neutral and nonreactionary way at certain points during the interview because of my emotional response to the content or Alexa's emotions. I found it challenging to balance rapport and impartiality at times.

Privacy was ensured throughout the process as directed by the course faculty and the informed consent. Alexa and I spoke to each other only in private or via telephone or e-mail. Neither of us indicated to others in our environment that the interviews had occurred.

The interview transcription analysis was tedious and long. The person analyzing the transcript needs time, patience, and, again, skill to disseminate the interview results as accurately as possible. The interviewer is the best person to complete this process, as he or she is present during the interview and is the most likely person to understand the interviewee's perceptions. The use of follow-up questions for clarification and understanding is helpful.

What I Would Do Differently

The next time I interview an individual or group of individuals, my objective will be to gain practice and experience before attempting such a large project. Although this interview did provide me with experience and clarity regarding the process, I felt that my interviewing skills were mediocre at best. In my profession, I have developed the ability to interview people and to look for nonverbal behaviors, but mostly for the person's medical and social history. I feel that I need more information on, and experience (even observing an experienced person) in, qualitative interviewing.

As much as I attempted to be objective during this interview, there were points when I was emotionally affected by what the interviewee was imparting. Learning to be more detached from the interviewee was difficult, as I am a caring person, and because I was familiar with the person.

I hope to improve as an interviewer as I gain exposure to and practice in interviewing for qualitative research. Whether it is research on an individual life history or human group life, qualitative research in nursing is expanding and increasing in popularity. Nursing is a caring and compassionate profession that is constantly looking for meaning and understanding as fundamentals to the practice of nursing (Munhill, 2012).The world consists of many perceptions of reality, and the qualitative researcher seeks to gain an understanding of the human experience.

REFERENCES

Denzin, N. K., & Lincoln, Y. S. (Eds.). (2005). *The sage handbook of qualitative research* (3rd ed.).Thousand Oaks, CA: Sage.

McEwen, M., & Wills, E. M. (2011). *Theoretical basis for nursing* (3rd ed.). Philadelphia, PA: Wolters Kluwer/Lippincott Williams & Wilkins.

Munhill, P. L. (2012). *Nursing research, a qualitative approach* (5th ed.). Sudbury, MA: Jones & Bartlett Learning.

LIST OF JOURNALS THAT PUBLISH QUALITATIVE RESEARCH

Mary de Chesnay

Conducting excellent research and not publishing the results negates the study and prohibits anyone from learning from the work. Therefore, it is critical that qualitative researchers disseminate their work widely, and the best way to do so is through publication in refereed journals. The peer review process, although seemingly brutal at times, is designed to improve knowledge by enhancing the quality of literature in a discipline. Fortunately, the publishing climate has evolved to the point where qualitative research is valued by editors and readers alike, and many journals now seek out, or even specialize in publishing, qualitative research.

The following table was compiled partially from the synopsis of previous work identifying qualitative journals by the St. Louis University Qualitative Research Committee (2013), with a multidisciplinary faculty, who are proponents of qualitative research. Many of these journals would be considered multidisciplinary, though marketed to nurses. All are peer reviewed. Other journals were identified by the author of this series and by McKibbon and Gadd (2004) in their quantitative analysis of qualitative research. It is not meant to be exhaustive, and we would welcome any suggestions for inclusion.

An additional resource is the nursing literature mapping project conducted by Sherwill-Navarro and Allen (Allen, Jacobs, & Levy, 2006). The 217 journals were listed as a resource for libraries to accrue relevant journals, and many of them publish qualitative research. Readers are encouraged to view the websites for specific journals that might be interested in publishing their studies. Readers are also encouraged to look outside the traditional nursing journals, especially if their topics more closely match the journal mission of related disciplines.

NURSING JOURNALS

Journal	Website
Advances in Nursing Science	www.journals.lww.com/advancesinnursingscience/pages/default.aspx
Africa Journal of Nursing and Midwifery	www.journals.co.za/ej/ejour_ajnm.html
Annual Review of Nursing Research	www.springerpub.com/product/07396686#.Uea Xbjvvv6U
British Journal of Nursing	www.britishjournalofnursing.com
Canadian Journal of Nursing Research	www.cjnr.mcgill.ca
Hispanic Health Care International	www.springerpub.com/product/15404153#.Uea X7jvvv6U
Holistic Nursing Practice	www.journals.lww.com/hnpjournal/pages/default.aspx
International Journal of Mental Health Nursing	www.onlinelibrary.wiley.com/journal/10.1111/(ISSN)1447-0349
International Journal of Nursing Practice	www.onlinelibrary.wiley.com/journal/10.1111/(ISSN)1440-172X
International Journal of Nursing Studies	www.journals.elsevier.com/international-journal-of-nursing-studies
Journal of Advanced Nursing	www.onlinelibrary.wiley.com/journal/10.1111/(ISSN)1365-2648
Journal of Clinical Nursing	www.onlinelibrary.wiley.com/journal/10.1111/(ISSN)1365-2702
Journal of Family Nursing	www.jfn.sagepub.com
Journal of Nursing Education	www.healio.com/journals/JNE
Journal of Nursing Scholarship	www.onlinelibrary.wiley.com/journal/10.1111/(ISSN)1547-5069
Nurse Researcher	www.nurseresearcher.rcnpublishing.co.uk
Nursing History Review	www.aahn.org/nhr.html
Nursing Inquiry	www.onlinelibrary.wiley.com/journal/10.1111/(ISSN)1440-1800
Nursing Research	www.ninr.nih.gov
Nursing Science Quarterly	www.nsq.sagepub.com
Online Brazilian Journal of Nursing	www.objnursing.uff.br/index.php/nursing

(continued)

Journal	Website
The Online Journal of Cultural Competence in Nursing and Healthcare	www.ojccnh.org
Public Health Nursing	www.onlinelibrary.wiley.com/journal/10.1111 /(ISSN)1525-1446
Qualitative Health Research	www.qhr.sagepub.com
Qualitative Research in Nursing and Healthcare	www.wiley.com/WileyCDA/WileyTitle/product Cd-1405161221.html
Research and Theory for Nursing Practice	www.springerpub.com/product/15416577#.Ueab lTvvv6U
Scandinavian Journal of Caring Sciences	www.onlinelibrary.wiley.com/journal/10.1111 /(ISSN)1471-6712
Western Journal of Nursing Research	http://wjn.sagepub.com

REFERENCES

Allen, M., Jacobs, S. K., & Levy, J. R. (2006). Mapping the literature of nursing: 1996–2000. *Journal of the Medical Library Association, 94*(2), 206–220. Retrieved from http://nahrs.mlanet.org/home/images/activity/nahrs2012selectedlist nursing.pdf

McKibbon, K., & Gadd, C. (2004). A quantitative analysis of qualitative studies in clinical journals for the publishing year 2000. *BMC Med Inform Decision Making, 4*, 11. Retrieved from http://www.ncbi.nlm.nih.gov/pmc/articles/PMC503397

St. Louis University Qualitative Research Committee. Retrieved July 14, 2013, from http://www.slu.edu/organizations/qrc/QRjournals.html

ESSENTIAL ELEMENTS FOR A QUALITATIVE PROPOSAL

Tommie Nelms

1. Introduction: Aim of the study
   a. Phenomenon of interest, and focus of inquiry
   b. Justification for studying the phenomenon (how big an issue/problem?)
   c. Phenomenon discussed within a specific context (lived experience, culture, human response)
   d. Theoretical framework(s)
   e. Assumptions, biases, experiences, intuitions, and perceptions related to the belief that inquiry into a phenomenon is important (researcher's relationship to the topic)
   f. Qualitative methodology chosen, with rationale
   g. Significance to nursing (How will the new knowledge gained benefit patients, nursing practice, nurses, society, etc.?)
   Note: The focus of interest/inquiry and statement of purpose of the study should appear at the top of page 3 of the proposal
2. Literature review: What is known about the topic? How has it been studied in the past?
   Include background of the theoretical framework and how it has been used in the past.
3. Methodology
   a. Introduction of methodology (philosophical underpinnings of the method)
   b. Rationale for choosing the methodology
   c. Background of methodology
   d. Outcome of methodology
   e. Methods: general sources, and steps and procedures
   f. Translation of concepts and terms

4. Methods
   a. Aim
   b. Participants
   c. Setting
   d. Gaining access, and recruitment of participants
   e. General steps in conduct of study (data gathering tool(s), procedures, etc.)
   f. Human subjects' considerations
   g. Expected timetable
   h. Framework for rigor, and specific strategies to ensure rigor
   i. Plans and procedures for data analysis

WRITING QUALITATIVE RESEARCH PROPOSALS

Joan L. Bottorff

PURPOSE OF A RESEARCH PROPOSAL

- Communicates research plan to others (e.g., funding agencies)
- Serves as a detailed plan of action
- Serves as a contract between investigator and funding bodies when proposal is approved

QUALITATIVE RESEARCH: BASIC ASSUMPTIONS

- Reality is complex, constructed, and, ultimately, subjective.
- Research is an interpretative process.
- Knowledge is best achieved by conducting research in the natural setting.

QUALITATIVE RESEARCH

- Qualitative research is unstructured.
- Qualitative designs are "emergent" rather than fixed.
- The results of qualitative research are unpredictable. (Morse, 1994)

KINDS OF QUALITATIVE RESEARCH

- Grounded theory
- Ethnography (critical ethnography, institutional ethnography, ethno-methodology, ethnoscience, etc.)
- Phenomenology
- Narrative inquiry
- Others

CHALLENGES FOR QUALITATIVE RESEARCHERS

- Developing a solid, convincing argument that the study contributes to theory, research, practice, and/or policy (the "so what?" question)
- Planning a study that is systematic, manageable, and flexible (to reassure skeptics):
  - Justification of the selected qualitative method
  - Explicit details about design and methods, without limiting the project's evolution
  - Attention to criteria for the overall soundness or rigor of the project

QUESTIONS A PROPOSAL MUST ANSWER

- Why should anyone be interested in my research?
- Is the research design credible, achievable, and carefully explained?
- Is the researcher capable of conducting the research? (Marshall & Rossman, 1999)

TIPS TO ANSWER THESE QUESTIONS

- Be practical (practical problems cannot be easily brushed off)
- Be persuasive ("sell" your proposal)
- Make broad links (hint at the wider context)
- Aim for crystal clarity (avoid jargon, assume nothing, explain everything) (Silverman, 2000)

SECTIONS OF A TYPICAL QUALITATIVE PROPOSAL

- Introduction
  - Introduction of topic and its significance
  - Statement of purpose, research questions/objectives
- Review of literature
  - Related literature and theoretical traditions
- Design and methods
  - Overall approach and rationale
  - Sampling, data gathering methods, data analysis
  - Trustworthiness (soundness of the research)
  - Ethical considerations
- Dissemination and knowledge translation
  - Timeline
  - Budget
  - Appendices

INTRODUCING THE STUDY—FIRST PARA

- Goal: Capture interest in the study
  - Focus on the importance of the study (Why bother with the question?)
  - Be clear and concise (details will follow)
  - Provide a synopsis of the primary target of the study
  - Present persuasive logic backed up with factual evidence

THE PROBLEM/RESEARCH QUESTION

- The problem can be broad, but it must be specific enough to convince others that it is worth focusing on.
- Research questions must be clearly delineated.
- The research questions must sometimes be delineated with sub-questions.
- The scope of the research question(s) needs to be manageable within the time frame and context of the study.

PURPOSE OF THE QUALITATIVE STUDY

- Discovery?
- Description?
- Conceptualization (theory building)?
- Sensitization?
- Emancipation?
- Other?

LITERATURE REVIEW

- The literature review should be selective and persuasive, building a case for what is known or believed, what is missing, and how the study fits in.
- The literature is used to demonstrate openness to the complexity of the phenomenon, rather than funneling toward an a priori conceptualization.

METHODS—CHALLENGES HERE

- Quantitative designs are often more familiar to reviewers.
- Qualitative researchers have a different language.

METHODS SECTION

- Orientation to the Method:
  - Description of the particular method that will be used and its creators/interpreters
  - Rationale for qualitative research generally and for the specific method to be used.

QUALITATIVE STUDIES ARE VALUABLE FOR RESEARCH

- It delves deeply into complexities and processes.
- It focuses on little-known phenomena or innovative systems.

- It explores informal and unstructured processes in organizations.
- It seeks to explore where and why policy and local knowledge and practice are at odds.
- It is based on real, as opposed to stated, organizational goals.
- It cannot be done experimentally for practical or ethical reasons.
- It requires identification of relevant variables. (Marshall & Rossman, 1999)

SAMPLE

- Purposive or theoretical sampling
  - The purpose of the sampling
  - Characteristics of potential types of persons, events, or processes to be sampled
  - Methods of making decisions about sampling
- Sample size
  - Estimates provided based on previous experience, pilot work, etc.
- Access and recruitment

DATA COLLECTION AND ANALYSIS

- Types: Individual interviews, participant observation, focus groups, personal and public documents, Internet-based data, videos, and so on, all of which vary with different traditions.
- Analysis methods vary depending on the qualitative approach.
- Add DETAILS and MORE DETAILS about how data will be gathered and processed (procedures should be made public).

QUESTIONS FOR DATA MANAGEMENT AND ANALYSIS

- How will data be kept organized and retrievable?
- How will data be "broken up" to see something new?
- How will the researchers engage in reflexivity (e.g., be self-analytical)?
- How will the reader be convinced that the researcher is sufficiently knowledgeable about qualitative analysis and has the necessary skills?

TRUSTWORTHINESS (SOUNDNESS OF THE RESEARCH)

- Should be reflected throughout the proposal
- Should be addressed specifically, with the relevant criteria for the qualitative approach used
- Should provide examples of the strategies used:
  - Triangulation
  - Prolonged contact with informants, including continuous validation of data
  - Continuous checking for representativeness of data and fit between coding categories and data
  - Use of expert consultants

EXAMPLES OF STRATEGIES FOR LIMITING BIAS IN INTERPRETATIONS

- Planning to search for negative cases
- Describing how analysis will include a purposeful examination of alternative explanations
- Using members of the research team to critically question the analysis
- Planning to conduct an audit of data collection and analytic strategies

OTHER COMPONENTS

- Ethical considerations
  - Consent forms
  - Dealing with sensitive issues
- Dissemination and knowledge translation
- Timeline
- Budget justification

LAST BITS OF ADVICE

- Seek assistance and pre-review from others with experience in grant writing. (plan time for rewriting)
- Highlight match between your proposal and purpose of competition.
- Follow the rules of the competition.
- Write for a multidisciplinary audience.

REFERENCES

Marshall, C., & Rossman, G. B. (1999). *Designing qualitative research*. Thousand Oaks, CA: Sage.

Morse, J. M. (1994). Designing funded qualitative research. In N. Denzin & Y. Lincoln (Eds.), *Handbook of qualitative research* (pp. 220–235). Thousand Oaks, CA: Sage.

Silverman, D. (2000). *Doing qualitative research*. Thousand Oaks, CA: Sage.

OUTLINE FOR A RESEARCH PROPOSAL

Mary de Chesnay

The following guidelines are meant as a general set of suggestions that supplement the instructions for the student's program. In all cases where there is conflicting advice, the student should be guided by the dissertation chair's instructions. The outlined plan includes five chapters: the first three constitute the proposal and the remaining two the results and conclusions, but the number may vary depending on the nature of the topic or the style of the committee chair (e.g., I do not favor repeating the research questions at the beginning of every chapter, but some faculty do. I like to use this outline but some faculty prefer a different order. Some studies lend themselves to four instead of five chapters.).

Chapter I: Overview of the Study (or Preview of Coming Attractions) is a few pages that tell the reader:

- What he or she is going to investigate (purpose or statement of the problem and research questions or hypotheses)
- What theoretical support the idea has (conceptual framework or theoretical support). In qualitative research, this section may include only a rationale for conducting the study, with the conceptual framework or typology emerging from the data.
- What assumptions underlie the problem
- What definitions of terms are important to state (typically, these definitions in quantitative research are called *operational definitions* because they describe how one will know the item when one sees it. An operational definition usually starts with the phrase: "a score of ... or above on the [name of instrument]"). One may also want to include a conceptual definition, which is the usual meaning of the concept of interest or a definition according to a specific author. In contrast, qualitative research usually does not include measurements, so operational definitions are not appropriate, but conceptual definitions may be important to state.

- What limitations to the design are expected (not delimitations, which are intentional decisions about how to narrow the scope of one's population or focus)
- What the importance of the study (significance) is to the discipline

Chapter II: The Review of Research Literature (or Why You Are Not Reinventing the Wheel)

For Quantitative Research:

Organize this chapter according to the concepts in the conceptual framework in Chapter I and describe the literature review thoroughly first, followed by the state of the art of the literature and how the study fills the gaps in the existing literature. Do not include non-research literature in this section—place it in Chapter I as introductory material if the citation is necessary to the description.

- Concept 1: a brief description of each study reviewed that supports concept 1 with appropriate transitional statements between paragraphs
- Concept 2: a brief description of each study reviewed that supports concept 2 with appropriate transitional statements between paragraphs
- Concept 3: a brief description of each study reviewed that supports concept 3 with appropriate transitional statements between paragraphs
- And so on, for as many concepts as there are in the conceptual framework (I advise limiting the number of concepts for a master's degree thesis owing to time and cost constraints)
- Areas of agreement in the literature—a paragraph, or two, that summarizes the main points on which authors agree
- Areas of disagreement—where the main issues on which authors disagree are summarized
- State of the art on the topic—a few paragraphs in which the areas where the literature is strong and where the gaps are, are clearly articulated
- A brief statement of how the study fills the gaps or why the study needs to be conducted to replicate what someone else has done

For Qualitative Research:

The literature review is usually conducted after the results are analyzed and the emergent concepts are known. The literature may then be placed in Chapter II of the proposal as shown earlier or incorporated into the results and discussion.

Chapter III: Methodology (or Exactly What You Are Going to Do Anyway)

- Design (name the design—e.g., ethnographic, experimental, survey, cross-sectional, phenomenological, grounded theory, etc.)
- Sample—describe the number of people who will serve as the sample and the sampling method: Where and how will the sample be recruited? Provide the rationale for sample selection and methods. Include the institutional review board (IRB) statement and say how the rights of subjects (Ss) will be protected, including how informed consent will be obtained and the data coded and stored.
- Setting—where will data collection take place? In quantitative research, this might be a laboratory or, if a questionnaire, a home. If qualitative, there are special considerations of privacy and comfortable surroundings for the interviews.
- Instruments and data analysis—how will the variables of interest be measured and how will sense be made of the data, if quantitative, and if qualitative, how will the data be coded and interpreted—that is, for both, this involves how the data will be analyzed.
- Validity and reliability—how will it be known if the data are good (in qualitative research, these terms are "accuracy" and "replicability").
- Procedures for data collection and analysis: a 1-2-3 step-by-step plan for what will be done
- Timeline—a chart that lists the plan month by month—use Month 1, 2, 3 instead of January, February, March.

The above three-chapter plan constitutes an acceptable proposal for a research project. The following is an outline for the final two chapters.

Chapter IV: Results (What I Discovered)

- Some researchers like to describe the sample in this section as a way to lead off talking about the findings.
- In the order of each hypothesis or research question, describe the data that addressed that question. Use raw data only; do not conclude anything about the data and make no interpretations.

Chapter V: Discussion (or How I Can Make Sense of All This)

- Conclusions—a concise statement of the answer to each research question or hypothesis. Some people like to interpret here—that is, to say how confident they can be about each conclusion.

- Implications—how each conclusion can be used to help address the needs of vulnerable populations or nursing practice, education, or administration.
- Recommendations for further research—that is, what will be done for an encore?

Index